GOODBYE MR. PRESIDENT

The story of one man's search for peace!
By Salem Kirban / Author of "I Predict"

GLENCAIRN
BAPTIST CHURCH
LIBRARY

First Printing .... December 1967
Second Printing .... January 1968
Third Printing .... January 1971
Fourth Printing .... July 1974

Published by SALEM KIRBAN Publishers, Kent Road, Huntingdon Valley, Penna. 19006 Copyright © 1967, 1974 by Salem Kirban. Printed in the United States of America. All rights reserved, including the right to reproduce this book or portions thereof in any form.

Library of Congress Catalog Card No. 67-31531
ISBN 0-912582-17-0

> At the daily 5 PM briefing to newsmen, casualties were described as "light" . . . 36 Americans killed in sporadic action.
>
> It was just a statistic.
>
> Then I witnessed the reality of that statistic.
>
> As I passed the filled aluminum containers ready to fly back to the States, I read the tags affixed to each one. They were just names—statistics back home—casualties that were described by the top Army echelon as "light."
>
> But they didn't seem "light" to me.
>
> And for the first time—I wept!

COVER PHOTO: Aluminum transfer cases are stacked up in a Vietnam area, ready for their grim task of returning Americans killed in the war.

"Some others are eager to enlarge the conflict. They call upon us to supply American boys to do what Asian boys should."

President Johnson

(In speech to American Bar Association on August 12, 1964)

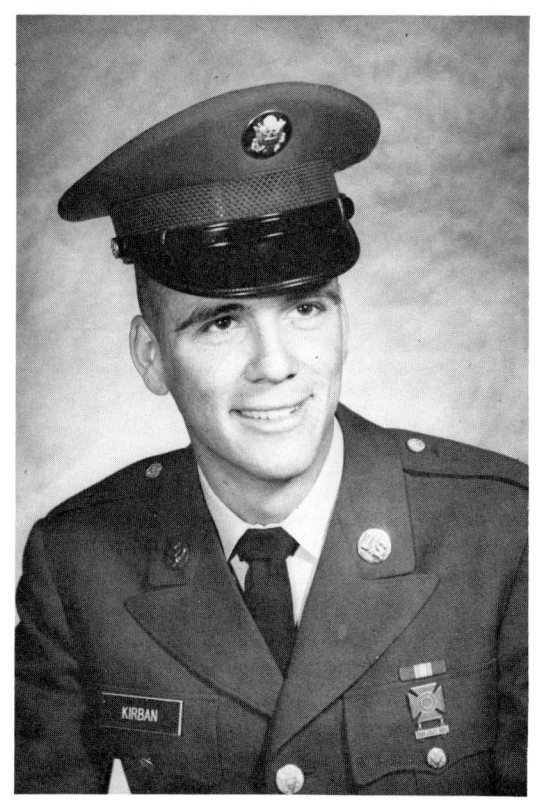

DENNIS KIRBAN

DEDICATED

First, to my wife, **Mary,** without whose loving understanding this trip would not have been possible . . .

to our son **Dennis,** whose service in Vietnam sparked the interest for this trip . . .

to our children, **Doreen, Diane, Duane and Dawn** . . . who originally suggested the idea . . .

and to THE PRESIDENT of the UNITED STATES, whose refusal to grant an ordinary citizen a private interview, generated a personal round-the-world fact-finding tour.

GOODBYE, MR. PRESIDENT

It was sunset! And the giant airliner was approaching San Francisco.

It was the first leg of an unusual journey . . . a journey which began 21 years ago and now was coming full circle.

I was a youngster then, fresh out of school—Girard College, a school for fatherless boys.

World War II was in full swing. And within a few months after graduation I was drafted into the U.S. Navy.

I'll never forget the day I climbed a hill overlooking the bay in Tsingtao, China. I was homesick. And as I watched the sun set over the ocean, I could picture it rising in Philadelphia.

How I longed to be with my sweetheart. We had our very first date the day I was inducted. And now I was engaged in a World War—a war all of us hoped would resolve into a permanent peace.

It would be hard to describe the thrill when our ship finally did return to the United States.

As we steamed under the Golden Gate bridge, we jumped for joy, tossing our white hats in the air. And when we hit land, many of us kissed the ground.

We were home.

But when I went to San Francisco, 21 years later it was like reliving my life.

This time the script was different. And my first day would be a day I would never forget.

How did this return voyage come about?

It started quite nonchalantly at our dinner table one evening.

My wife, Mary, and four of our children, Doreen, Diane, Duane, and Dawn were discussing the war in Vietnam. We had a personal interest in it. For in November, 1966 our son had enlisted in the Army.

And within six months he was in Vietnam.

The myth of World War II being a war to end all wars had vanished, for 21 years later, my son was returning to the same war zone to which our AKA35 Cargo Transport ship had sailed.

At the dinner table we talked about the war. I was fortunate enough to visit my son in basic training at Fort Gordon, Georgia and at advance training in Fort Huachuca, Arizona.

Then one of our children spoke up, "Daddy, why don't you go to Vietnam?" It was a rather startling question. I was about to dismiss it with a casual answer. Such a trip would be impossible, I thought.

After all, the Government knows more about the war than I do. What could I hope to accomplish in a few weeks in the war zone that they couldn't accomplish in many years of conflict?

The Government—I thought—am I not the Government?

I had always thought of the Government as that impersonal body in Washington that took care of everything. Now I just wasn't sure they were doing a good job.

In effect, I, as an American citizen, had employed them to represent me. Wasn't it my right to check on their performance?

"Why don't you go to Vietnam, Daddy?"

"Well," I replied, "I'll write the President and ask him for a personal interview. Maybe he'll be able to answer some of my questions on this war, and that will save me a trip."

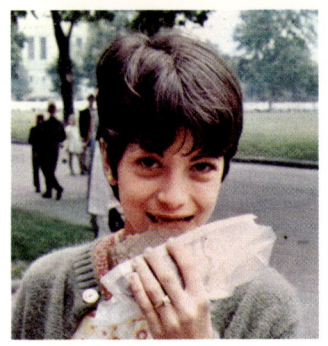

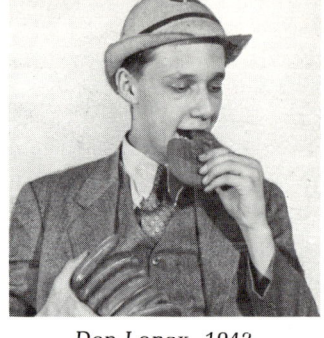

Doreen Kirban, 1968   Don Lenox, 1943

The Girard "Ginger" was the equivalent of money while the Author was in Girard College. A plump, oversize cookie, rich in nutrients and molasses, it was highly treasured...awarded for doing errands, etc. My classmate of June, 1943, Don Lenox, with 7 "Hum Muds," as they were affectionately called... could be considered extremely rich.

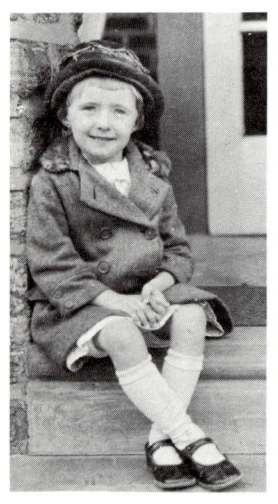

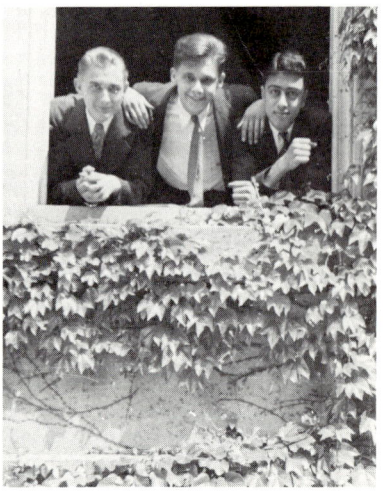

Photo at left of little girl was taken at 4300 N. 8th Street in Philadelphia in the early 1930's. For who she is...turn to page 163. Photo at right is the "Three Musketeers" at Girard College: Jim Cleaver, Don Lenox and Salem Kirban in 1943.

I wrote.

Back came a reply from Mr. Donald Ropa of the Defense Department of the White House. President Johnson was sorry, but his schedule could not permit a personal interview. Mr. Ropa, however, indicated he would be willing to answer my questions.

But when you're in love with a girl, just talking to her mother does not quite generate the same interest.

And having viewed poverty and disease-ridden countries in World War II, I had come back more in love with my country.

I wanted to talk to the man I appointed to represent me — my President.

Day Of Decision

Through the newspapers, radio and TV I had accumulated private opinions about the war in Vietnam, but I did not feel it fair to my President to voice these publicly or to take part in protest rallies or join peace marchers. I felt a responsibility to my country. And to me that responsibility negated such action.

It's easy to be either a protest marcher or a mere flag waver spouting patriotism. Neither takes any degree of intelligence, and just a fine line separate both.

Freedom carried to irresponsible extremes represented to me many of the doves, who unfortunately had an entourage of shaggy haired, unkempt youths.

And it also represented the emotional — almost to the point of hysteria — blind, vocal, super-patriot.

It's so easy to join either of these camps.

But's it's so much more difficult to be a responsible American citizen, earnestly trying to find workable solutions to peace that will bring honor to the United States and to the basic concepts on which it was founded.

I do not believe in the theory of America — right or wrong. No one can be perfect. I was distressed by some of the things our government had done for political expediency. Confession, they say, is good for the soul. And I believe when America makes a mistake it should admit it — and no

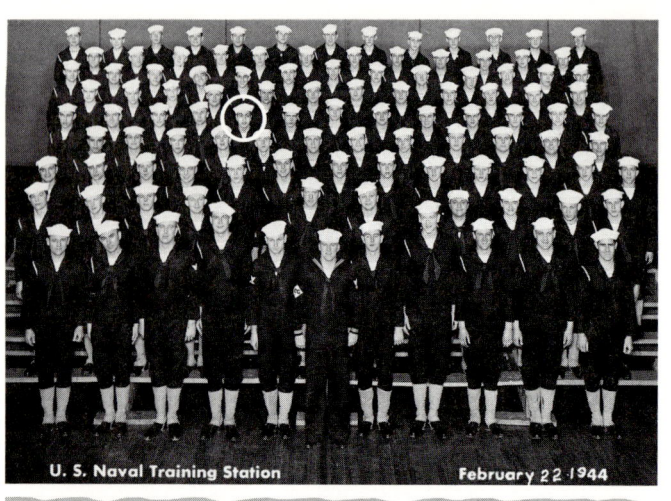

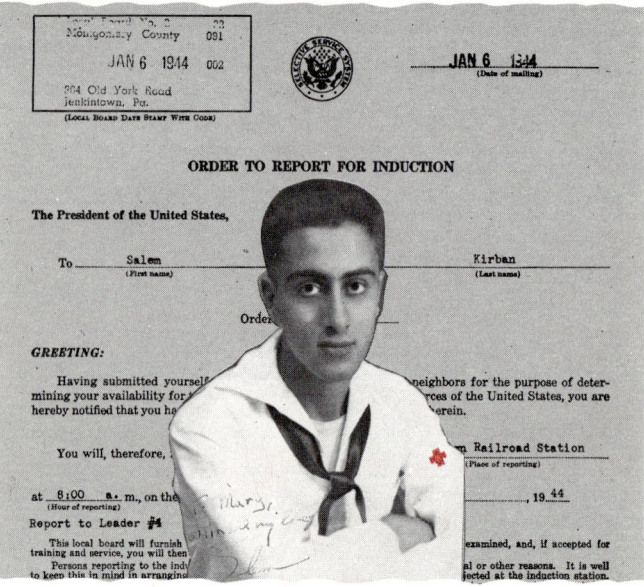

Top photo: Author's boot training picture at U.S. Naval Training Station in Sampson, New York.

Bottom: An invitation from the United States Government for the Author to join the Armed Forces on January 18, 1944.

American should have an irresponsible patriotism that condones such transgressions.

These preceding paragraphs have been related to explain my next move . . .

If my President could not see me, then, before I voiced any opinion on world conditions, I would make a trip around the world on my own private Fact-Finding Mission.

Sponsored by no one, paying my own expenses, I could report the facts as I viewed them first hand.

An Invitation To The President

When I approached a news man at the Washington Post regarding my trip to Vietnam, his question was. "Do you intend to accomplish in a few days what the government could not do in a few years?"

My reply was: "Do you think I have a right to sit back here in the United States and voice armchair opinions? Or should I view these conditions first hand before reflecting on U.S. policy?" "After all," I added, "sometimes government officials can be so close to the forest they can't see the trees."

I placed a fourteen inch ad in the Washington Post Wednesday, July 12, It was titled "Goodbye, Mr. President." In it I related my mission—how I intended to fly to riot-torn Hong Kong, war-torn Vietnam, Israel, Egypt and Jordan seeking solutions for world peace.

I invited him to send me off at the airport. I also requested he allow me personally to present him with my Private Citizen Report on world conditions and solutions to peace when I returned August 15.

The die was cast. What started as a question from a trusting child—"Daddy, why don't you go to Vietnam?" was now becoming a reality.

It was at the Army Processing Center in Oakland, California, that my son, Dennis, was processed for a flight to Vietnam.

And on the Sunday evening of July 16, I began the long journey—the journey of a concerned father following his son's footsteps.

As the plane touched down at San Francisco's International Airport, the sun disappeared over the horizon. Darkness was creeping in. And tomorrow would bring the stark revelations of the reality of war. It would be a day I would never forget.

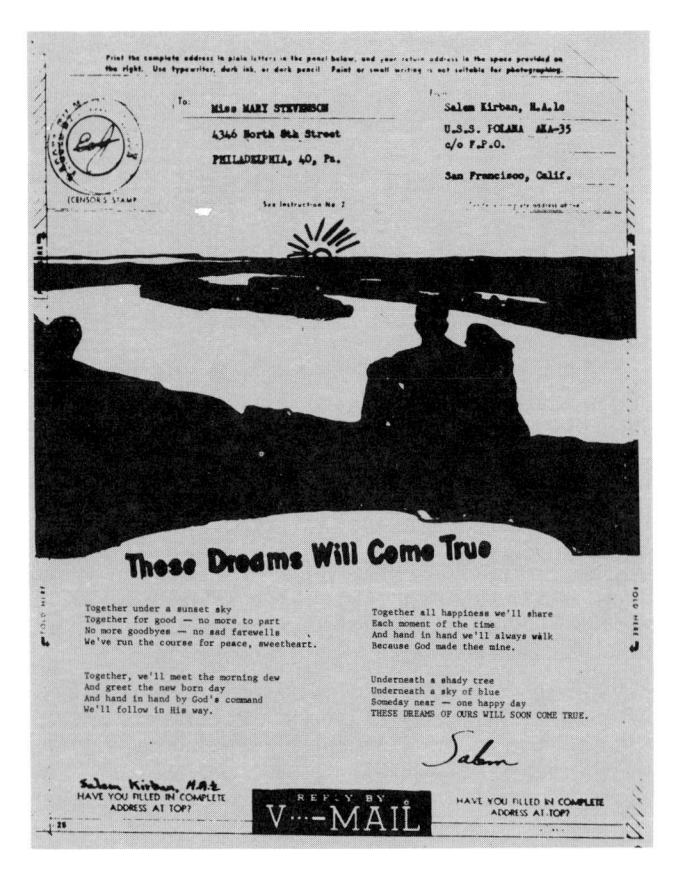

During World War 2, to save space, the War Department devised a miniaturized letter form known as V-mail. Above is V-mail letter Author sent to his sweetheart, Mary, while in the Pacific in 1945. V-mail letter's actual size was not much bigger than one pictured. And incidentally, our dreams have come true!

OAKLAND ARMY PROCESSING CENTER—AS I SAW IT

A Study in Contrasts

Sadness and joy, they say, are separated by only a fine line. I found this true at Oakland.

G.I.'s fresh from 21 days leave arrived daily at this giant Army base located near the waterfront. From the luxuries of home and a full shock of hair, the next few minutes quickly brought them back to the reality of their mission.

Open jitneys transported them around the base. And at the processing point they unloaded their heavy duffel bags in neat rows outside. Gloom and bewilderment prevailed.

They stood at attention while a sergeant barked orders. Then inside they march to an orientation room. As I witnessed this and other events of the day, my mind's eye tried to picture the discouragement that must have passed through my son's thoughts as he followed this procedure through this gloomy, cavernous building.

He had just become engaged and was experiencing, as I had experienced in World War II, the heartbreak of leaving a fiancé back home.

Before my personally conducted tour began, however, a courteous but tough warrant officer had to clear my itinerary. The Information Officer was called in San Francisco. And he in turn called Washington.

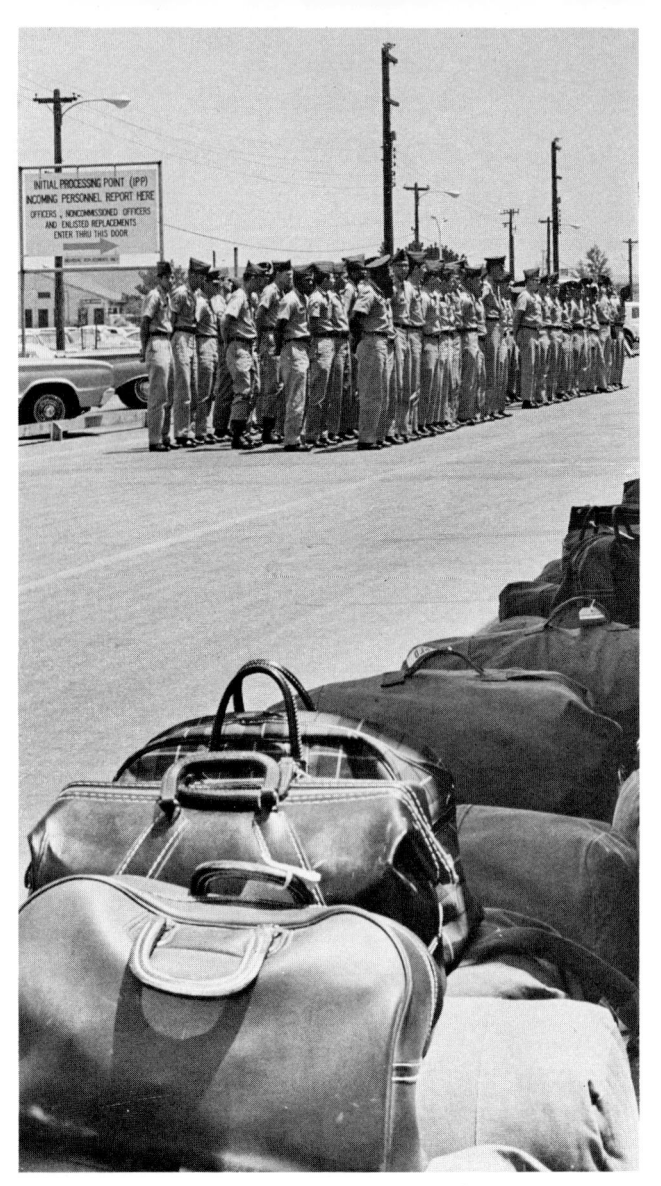

Fresh from leave, GI's lined up at Oakland Processing Center to begin the long journey to Vietnam.

Two hours after my arrival at 8:00 A.M., I was cleared and my tour began.

At the orientation room, G.I.'s outbound for Vietnam started the day-long procedure of going over. They were given pencils and forms. Here at Oakland they processed 600 to 700 soldiers a day. All those under 18 or who had a wife seven month's pregnant were asked to raise their hands. A directive from the Army prohibited those under 18 to enter the war zone. In the midst of the mechanical impersonal channeling of soldiers, here was one pause of compassion.

From orientation they proceeded to the verification counter where their orders and records were checked. If they needed money, pay was advanced them. Army policy provided that a serviceman going overseas should have at least $30 with him.

Those requiring immunization were given their final shots. Some got one or two—others need 4 or 5. And in less than a minute, they got them—in both arms.

The Thin Line Of Joy

Happiness and sadness are only a hairbreadth apart. Here at Oakland Processing Center, they were only a room apart. For while sad-eyed youngsters were being prepared for war in Vietnam, just a room away in the gym area, battle weary veterans were beginning the long-awaited trip home.

What a study in contrasts! Their bags, too, were neatly stacked in square painted blocks on the gym floor while they waited and waited and waited. Exhausted from their 18 hour flight from Vietnam, they were sprawled in all positions on hard wooden benches . . . that is, until a young Lieutenant walked in and barked orders for them to sit up.

One compensation they did receive, however, was that upon their arrival at Oakland—regardless of the hour— they were given a full course steak dinner.

While actual processing can be done in one day for the outgoing G.I., the inflow of traffic was so great a soldier remained at Oakland usually 3 to 5 days.

In contrast, these returning from Vietnam were processed out of Oakland and on the way home in 4-5 hours.

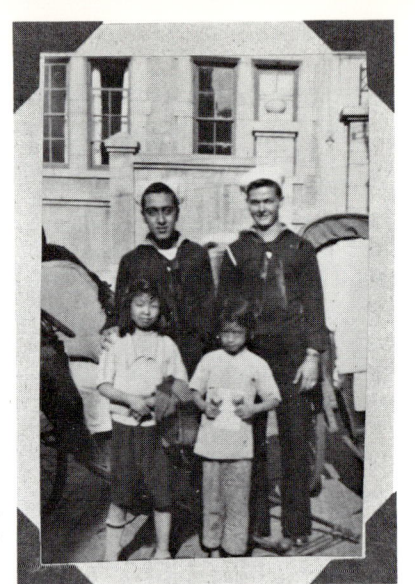

Seaman Anfinson with Hospital Corpsman Salem Kirban in Tsingtao, China, November 5, 1945. Note two Chinese rickshaws in background.

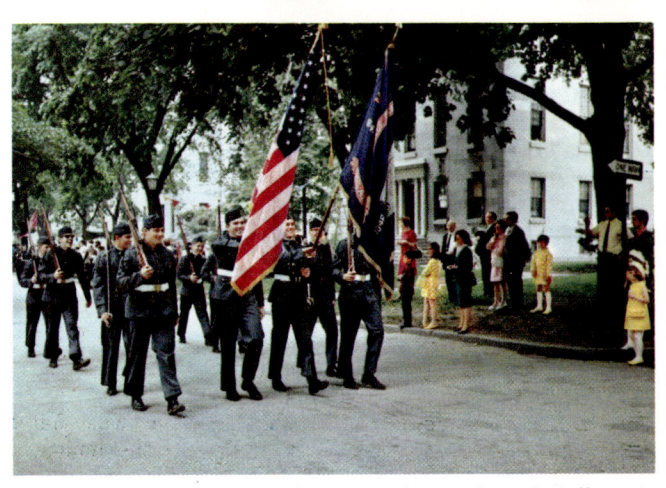

Author's military training began early...at Girard College in Philadelphia, actually an elementary and high school for fatherless boys. Every student who did not learn a musical instrument received one hour of military training every week. The Battalion is pictured in its annual Founder's Day march in May, 1968.

Once processing was completed, the soldier boarded a bus for the hour trip to Travis Air Force Base. Upon my arrival at Travis, I again had to receive security clearance from two or three sources. Travis is a huge complex of buildings, the flight center of the West, nestled among mountain ranges on a plateau of sand.

The airport terminal was bursting at the seams and construction was in progress to enlarge the facility.

Everywhere there were servicemen from all branches with their wives and dependents. There were also Vietnamese officers, trained in the United States, and returning to their homeland.

From 1965-1967 troop movements to Vietnam escalated to such a degree that the government contracted commercial carriers to aid in overseas flights.

A Study In Contrasts

And here again the study in contrast becomes evident.

On one apron a brightly painted yellow Braniff 707 loads troops bound for Vietnam—and just one apron away (300 feet) a giant windowless Army Transport plane unloads war veterans returning home after a year overseas.

And in the lobby there are tears of sadness as wives and sweethearts kiss their loved ones goodbye, not knowing whether this may be the last time they may ever see them alive—and a few steps away a mother, a wife is crying with tears of happiness as she embraces her son or husband after a year's separation.

Those servicemen fortunate enough to fly over or back on a commercially chartered airline, fly in comparative luxury with windows, pretty hostesses, and full-course hot meals.

Those less fortunate, fly in Air Force planes—no windows, seated so they are flying backwards, and served TV dinners by their fellow G.I.'s.

But these minor inconveniences of life are nothing to be compared to those who have become just another statistic.

Here again, the study of contrasts becomes increasingly evident, and sickening as well as tragic.

Returning servicemen arrive around the clock, but usually in daylight hours. I witnessed two incoming flights.

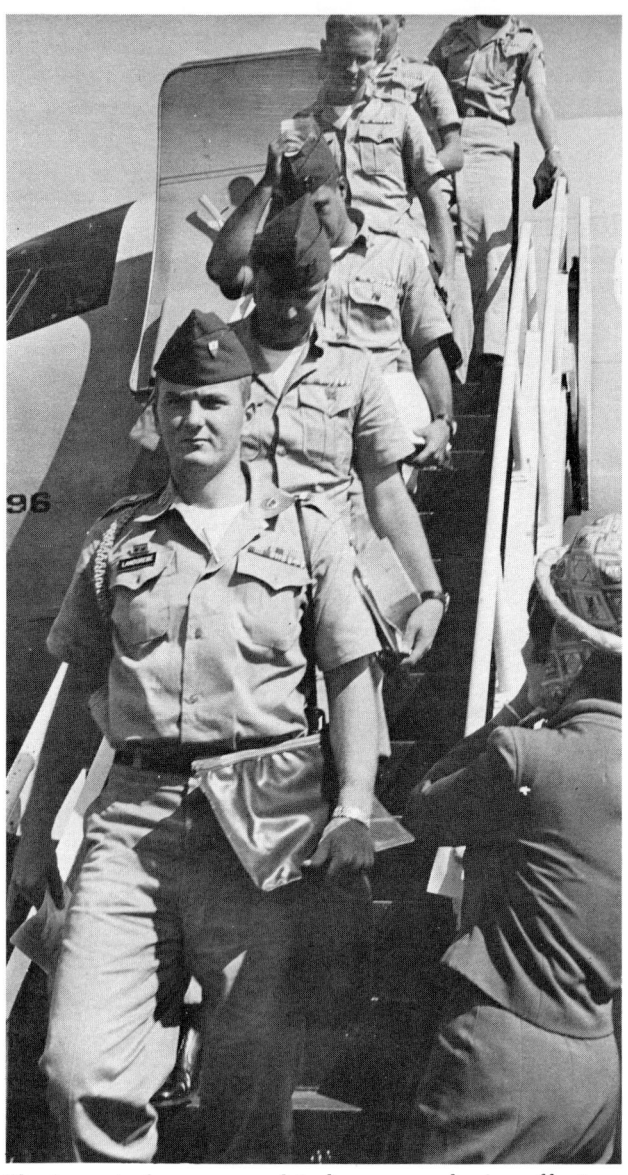

The impact of war seemed to have a sombering effect on GI's returning to the United States.

It was Monday afternoon, July 17, 1967. Not a cloud in the sky. The warm California sun basked the entire area in pleasant 80° weather.

The Air Force guide assigned to me, directed me right to the flight apron. I had my still and movie cameras with me and also a tape recorder. I asked him to tape-record the scene—the subsiding roar of the jet engines, the exuberant cheers, and exicted conversations of the returning servicemen.

I recalled that memorable day in 1946 when I returned. We jumped for joy, flung our hats in the air, kissed the ground. I recalled the calendar I sent my son. He told me how each day he marks off the calendar, anxious for the day he will return.

A Different War

And I wanted to capture this moment of joy both on film and on tape.

Everything was ready. The flight arrival steps were wheeled to the plane. The door opened. A customs officer entered the plane. One minute passed. Two minutes. The stewardess appeared. I flicked the tape recorder on and began my filming.

But the only sound I picked up was the rustle of the wind— a far off soft whine of a jet. My film recorded only the somber, expressionless faces of battle-weary men.

I was shocked.

"Was this the wrong plane?" I asked my guide. "Are these men coming home from Vietnam?"

"This is the right plane," he replied. "It's just come from Pleiku. But every incoming flight from Vietnam is the same. No overt joy, just quiet somberness. Somehow it's just a different war."

Under Cover Of Darkness

What about the wounded, I wondered? I wanted to see one of these planes land. I was told this was not practical. Wounded are usually flown into Travis from Vietnam on flight schedules geared to time their arrival here under cover of darkness.

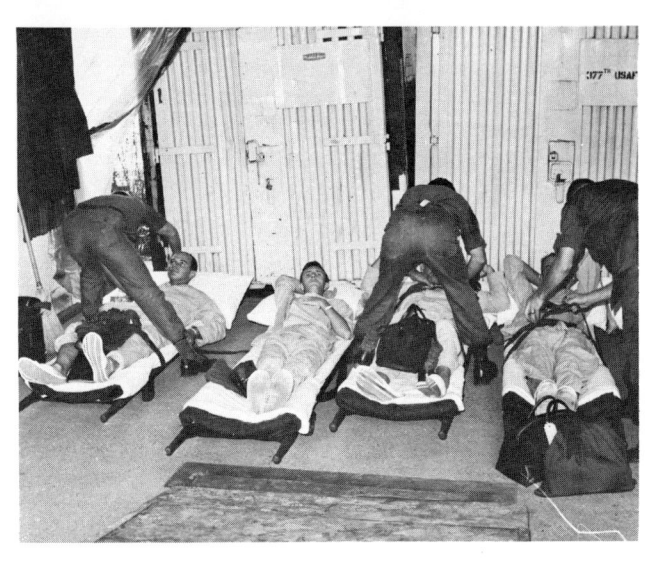

Casualties being readied for evacuation to hospitals.

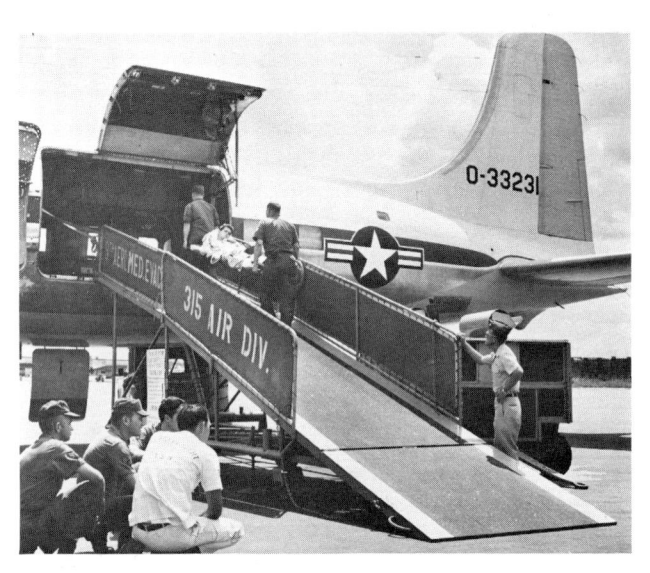

Medical Evacuation plane ferries seriously wounded to hospitals in Japan and the United States.

Specially constructed aircraft can accommodate about 50 such cases. The few that are ambulatory sit up front; the balance are on stretchers 4-tiered in the rear of the aircraft.

They are deplaned at a remote section of the airport, usually late at night or very early in the morning.

"And what about the dead?" I inquired.

I was told the government was a little touchy on the subject and further clearance would be required for me to view this area.

As I drove off the base, I purposely first took a little-noticed side road. It wound round and round to a remote area of flat barren land, dotted sporadically with low, one-story, inconspicuous buildings.

And there it was—a humble, small, mist-green building— about the size of a bungalow. No architectural beauty this —a simple severe rectangular building. A small sign read Mortuary—that's all.

A soldier stood guard. And the only sound I heard was the awesome thunder of silence.

And as I drove on, I noticed another building—this one slightly smaller. Previous contacts had alerted me that here was where unidentifiable servicemen were sent until positive identification could be made.

Joy and sadness—just a few feet apart. The bewilderment of the troops going to Vietnam, the restrained joy of battle-weary troops returning home, and the stark reality of war in the little green building buried away from the crowds where the thrill and glories of war somehow echo back into a sickening hollow ring!

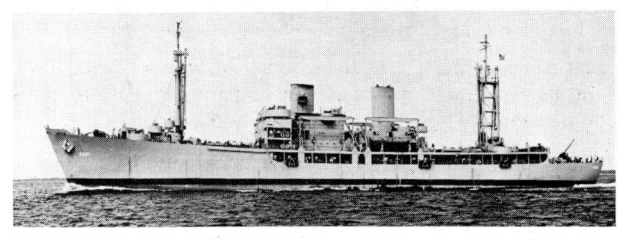

U.S.S. POLANA (AKA-35) on sea trial out of Walsh-Kaiser shipyards in Newport News, Rhode Island. This is the combat-cargo ship on which I served a year in the Pacific in 1944-45.

ESCORT SERVICE
WAR'S MOST TRAGIC TASK

Within a few steps from where medics were giving shots to Vietnam-bound soldiers was an enclosed office—about the size of a spacious living room. There was no welcome sign here, however.

Inside were two administrative personnel and the Captain of the Escort Service.

Outside the door was a padlock, and entrance was only gained by securing prior clearance. This was the office of the 6th U.S. Army Escort Unit.

Their mission was to provide trained escort personnel to accompany and insure safe delivery of remains of deceased military personnel to designated places of interment.

I was cleared to discuss the Escort Service with its Commanding Officer, Captain Bryan L. Nott, who in 10 days would complete his tour of service and return to the field of law.

The Sixth Army has the Army port responsibility for ferrying all remains that come from Southeast Asia to Continental United States terminating points.

A detachment of the Escort Service was located in Dover, Delaware. As much as possible, war dead who came from an area North and South of the Ohio River Valley and East of that area went to Dover, Delaware. All other war dead came to Travis Air Force Base, located about 30 miles from Sacramento, California.

Death Knows No Rank

The long road home began in Vietnam. Here bodies were shipped by Boeing 707 jets in vented aluminum containers to either Travis or Dover.

At this point the Escort Service began. Several guidelines were used to determine which escort would accompany each body.

First, the escort chosen is usually the same grade as the deceased. A lieutenant would accompany a lieutenant—a sergeant, a sergeant, etc.

Also in the selection of an escort, they try to choose one of the same religion and of the same language.

Only one person was assigned as escort for each body. The escort merely accompanies the remains, either to the funeral director or next of kin. There his responsibility ends. By request of kin, he can stay for the duration of the funeral if they so desire.

Escorts are highly selected. The escalation of the war in October, 1965, brought an increase in war dead. This resulted in the establishing of a permanent functioning Escort Service. The Sixth Army went out into the field and hand selected qualified volunteers. Most had either World War II or Korean War experience.

Periodic classes were held on the conduct and duties of an escort.

Further, each escort has a briefing prior to going to his mission of each particular case. Escort Command has provided service from privates on up to a general.

In each case, the escort learns the background of the individual he is escorting, and many times lasting friendships are born between the escort and loved ones of the deceased.

I asked Captain Nott how he scheduled his work load. His reply, "Just by the papers, we can almost forecast what our Escort requirements for next week will be. In World War II and Korea, it used to take some two weeks between the time a man was listed as killed in action to the time

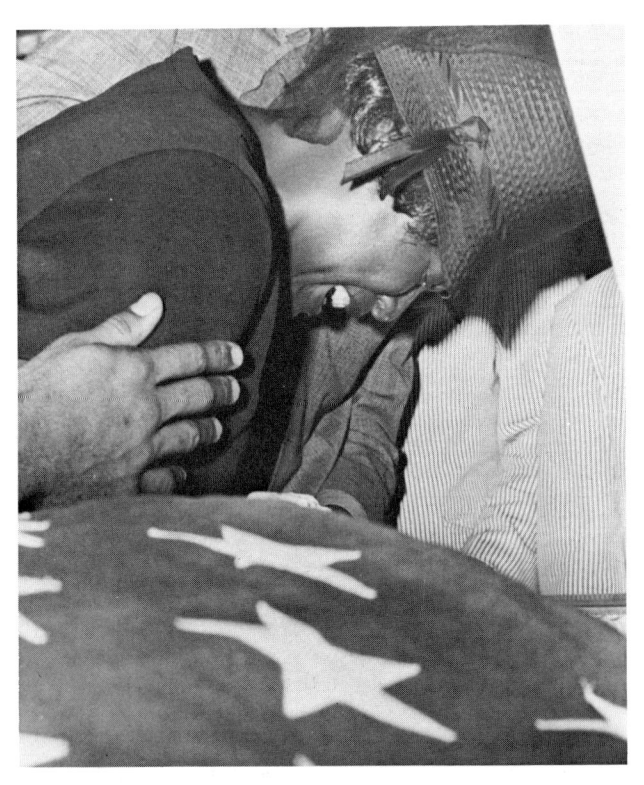

SON LOST

SP/4 Poindexteur Williams, killed in the Vietnam War, was denied burial in a Florida cemetery. The reason: because he was black. The funeral began with full military and religious honors at an armory in Fort Pierce, Florida. But when the coffin reached the white cemetery officials refused to accept it.

This photograph was dramatically taken at this point of refusal and shows Mrs. Mary Campbell weeping over her son's coffin.

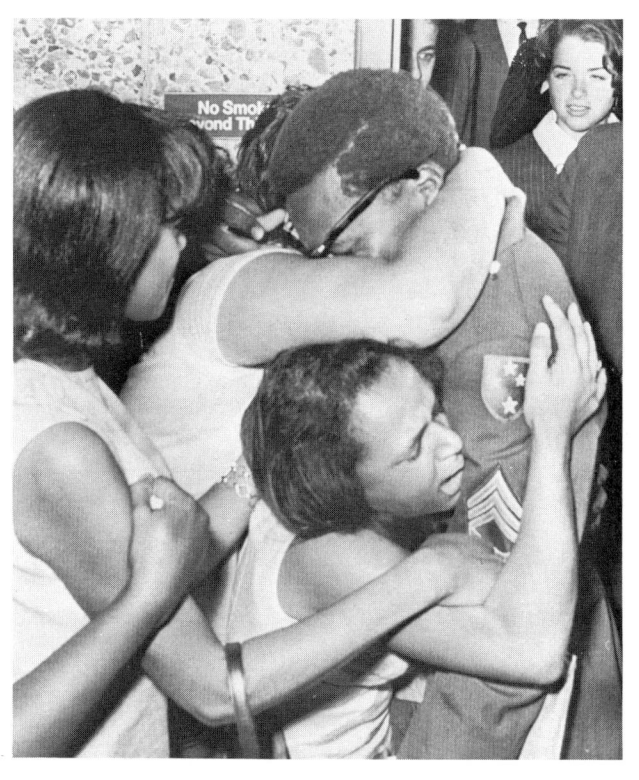

SON FOUND

Soldier returns from the dead. S/Sgt. James O. Williams is greeted by relatives as he arrived at airport in Detroit, Michigan on a 30-day leave. William's widowed mother had been notified by Army officers that her son had died in Vietnam. A telegram confirmed his death. But the next day Army authorities again called to report the Army had made a mistake!

he was interred in the United States, but now it takes only about 5 or 6 days.

The Army Command at Oakland had 52 escorts. It takes each escort about a week to fulfill his duty. The next of kin is allowed use of the escort for 72 hours for any help or assistance. The escort presents a flag to the next of kin.

Escorts have many unique experiences.

One escort sergeant was made an honorary citizen of New Mexico when he escorted a Medal of Honor winner back to his home state. He subsequently was summoned to the White House to accompany the parents for the presentation of the Medal of Honor by President Johnson.

After arrival at Travis, the remains were transported to a mortuary right at the Army Processing Center in Oakland, and here is where the escort begins his responsibility.

The job of an escort is a very sensitive one. Not only must he fulfill his responsibility, but also, many times, bear the brunt of animosity a grieving parent or wife has for the war. But in the majority of cases, he is treated as a member of the family—taken home for dinner and treated wonderfully.

"Outside of fighting," Captain Nott concluded, "escort duty is the most honorable service a soldier can perform."

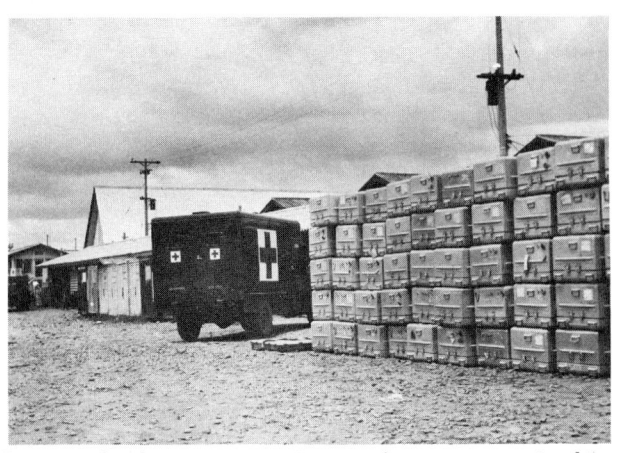

Over 50 dead servicemen, in transfer cases, await shipment from Vietnam back to the United States. Back home it would just be considered "another statistic."

JAPAN . . . . A NEW INSIGHT INTO THE WAR

From Oakland my son Dennis flew direct to Vietnam with stop-overs for refueling in Hawaii and Guam.

He arrived in Vietnam before his bags did and I recall him writing that he slept four days in the same clothes right on the ground.

We were all concerned where he would be stationed but we realized no station would be assigned until his bags were located.

When his bags finally arrived Dennis was shipped to Nha Trang—a coastal city in Vietnam about midway between Saigon and the DMZ.

When a youngster comes out of high school often one is not sure what vocation he wants to pursue. We wanted Dennis to go to college. But like many youngsters he was not interested. One of my businesses was wedding photography and I taught him the rudiments of the trade. But he could never generate interest in photography although he did learn the basics.

His main interest was cars and had three 15-20 year old models with which he was constantly puttering. He was adept at office work and his training at Fort Huachuca prepared him for this skill.

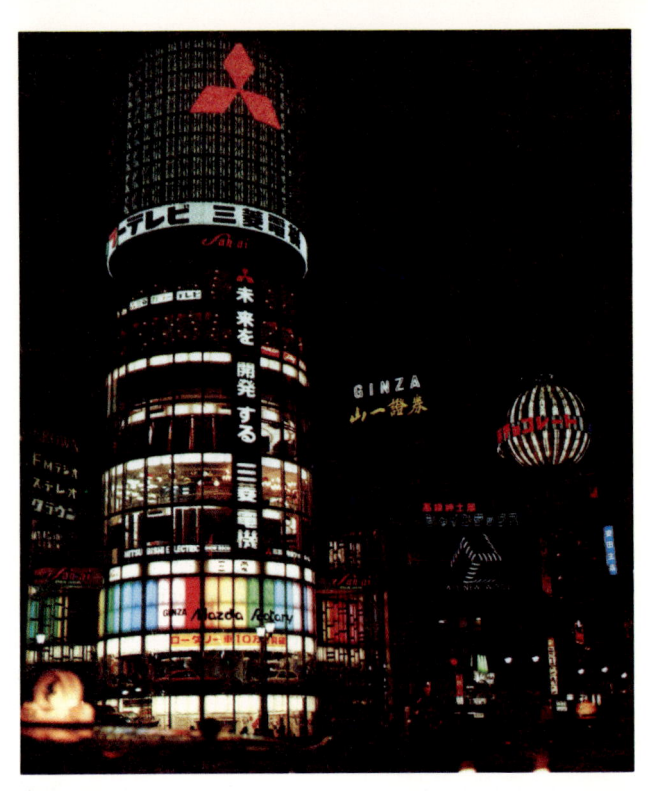

The Ginza...the downtown section of Tokyo...at night. Tokyo is the world's largest city with over 12 million people. Already in Tokyo there are 20,000 people living per square mile! To the city of Tokyo is being added 7000 tons of garbage a day to fill Tokyo bay. By the year 2000, 40 million people will be living in Tokyo!

Arriving in Nha Trang three men were competing for the same position at Headquarters Company—one a college graduate. Two of them would be sent out to field camps in less secure areas.

A decision was to be made—one that would show my son how valuable experience can be. The Information Officer was seeking someone with a background of photography. As a result the college graduate and other contender for the job ended up in field companies. Dennis was given the job of photography and reporting.

I'll never forget his letter in which he thanked me for training him in photography—a skill he hated but had now come to like.

His letters also revealed how he regretted not going to college. The privileges officers enjoy even in wartime made this fact increasingly evident.

Now that he was permanently assigned, his year overseas would begin. Since he was in a war zone there would be the benefits of extra pay but also extra hazards.

The United States had close to 500,000 Americans fighting the war in Vietnam. My son was one of them. Why was it, I wondered, that other countries in the Far East—who stand most to gain from the resolving of this conflict—were not themselves involved?

I was particularly concerned about Japan. Why weren't their soldiers lending support? With talk about even increasing U.S. manpower in Vietnam with more U.S. casualties—weren't we fighting a lopsided war?

With a fair spread of wartime responsibility among other nations my son and sons of perhaps a quarter million other Americans would not be engaged in the devasting consequences of war.

It is with this reason in mind that I decided to stop first in Japan en route to Vietnam.

It was a warm, sunny day when I arrived in Japan—this time as a friend.

The New Face Of Japan

Twenty-two years ago our ship had sailed into Yokohoma harbor as conquerors.

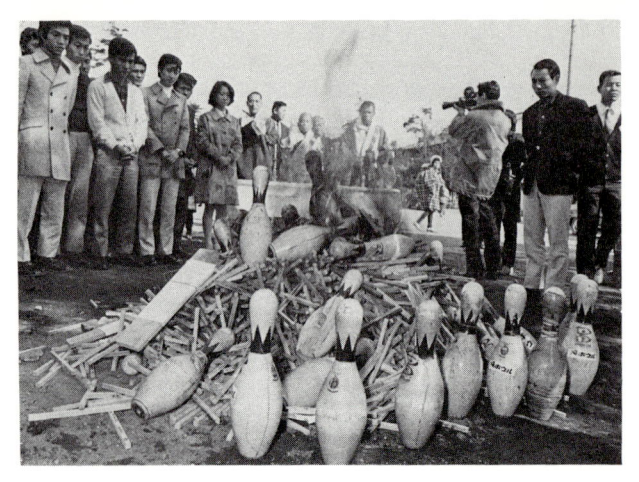

A buddhist worship service for departed bowling pins. While the bowling alley owners and staff are standing in reverence, a Buddhist priest chants prayers for the final rest of damaged bowling pins.

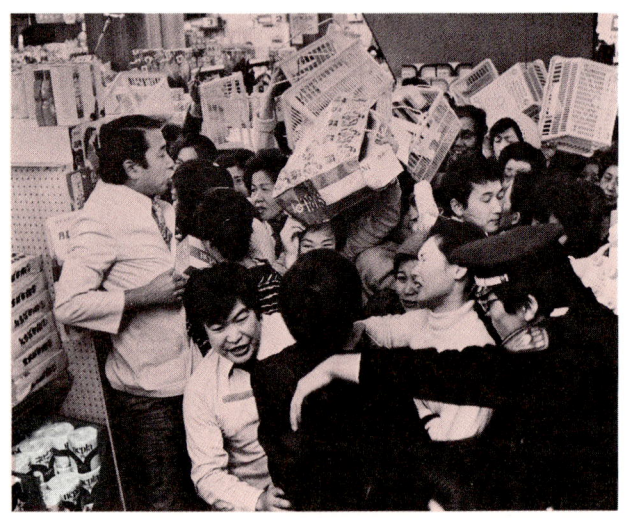

Increasing shortages have caused many Japanese housewives to panic in supermarkets in a determination to secure scarce items. In this case...the cause for the stampede is seen in the lower left of the photograph — toilet tissue!

Today I flew into Tokyo and it looked like New York City from the air. It's hard to realize that this city was two-thirds destroyed in World War II.

Several things immediately impressed me. The people were very courteous. So used to the impolite and dour personalities of many in the U.S., I was rather shocked at the bowing and extreme courtesy of bus and taxi drivers, bell hops, and store clerks. It was most refreshing, and I soon found my attitudes of courtesies changing.

Two days later I, too, was bowing and saying "Thank you."

Then, too, one can't help noticing the cleanliness of Tokyo. It's not unusual to see a cab driver or pedestrian stop to pick up a piece of paper. Many cars carry feather dusters, and cab drivers, while waiting for a passenger, often spend their time washing and waxing their cabs. It was with these pleasant observations that I hired a limousine for a day and went to the largest daily newspaper in Tokyo. I had not made a previous appointment. But after funneling my way through a series of officials, I was finally escorted to a private office.

Here I interviewed one of the top leaders of the Japanese Press. He requested, however, his name not be used.

The Japanese are very thorough, and he expressed surprise that I had not studied Japanese culture before I came to Japan. I replied that if I had wanted to learn more about my wife, I wouldn't spend time talking to her mother—and that while my stay in Japan was brief (only 2 days), I believed coming to Japan was better than studying about the country.

Bombs Make The Difference

This seemed to satisfy him and the interview began. It must be remembered that the views of the Japanese people are conditioned by World War II. Their suffering in the war was much greater than ours in that the United States soil was never bombed. Japan was devastated by bombs and was the recipient of two atomic bombs. In light of this, my understanding of their position was quite clear.

I had heard so much concerning the validity of our commitment to Asia that I asked this Japanese newsman: "Do you feel the war in Vietnam holds any security for Asia?"

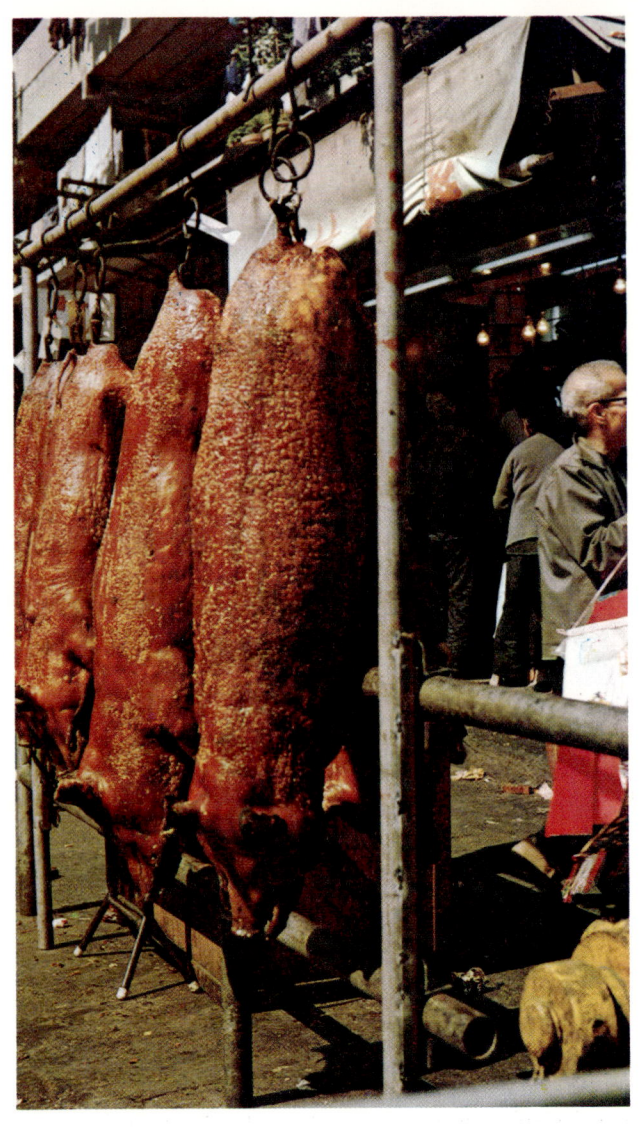

Open air butcher shop in Hong Kong.

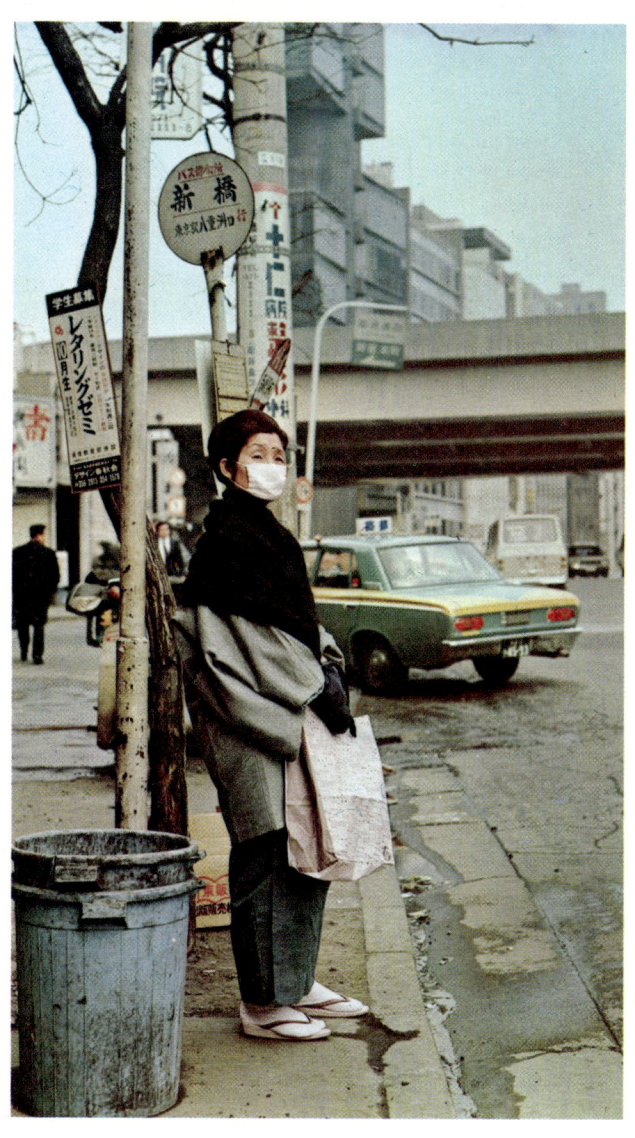

A common scene in Tokyo. To avoid disease germs and industrial pollutants some residents wear face masks.

LITTLE KNOWN FACTS about a WELL-KNOWN WAR

Many of our allies were profiting more from the war in Vietnam than they were contributing in aid.

While Japan has given Vietnam $2.2 million in aid since 1964 . . . in 1966 alone it profited $138 million in exports to Saigon.

From 1964 to 1966 Japan's trade with North Vietnam was about 20 times the amount of Japan's assistance to South Vietnam during the same period.

Italy's trade with North Vietnam was more than 10 times Italy's assistance to South Vietnam.

New Zealand's trade with North Vietnam was about 8 times its assistance to South Vietnam.

The Netherlands' trade with North Vietnam was more than 3 times its assistance to South Vietnam.

The United Kingdom's trade with North Vietnam was almost twice the amount of assistance to South Vietnam.

(Source: Senate Foreign Relations Committee)

His reply was quick: "No!"

"The Japanese," he continued "very much want to restore peace."

"Isn't it true," I asked, "that if we do not fight in Vietnam communism will spread?"

"No, this was an old conception, started I believe with Dulles. Indonesia, Burma, and India were all examples that this theory does not hold water. Americans may claim that the tide in the Vietnam war appeared to be in favor of the U.S., but actually the anti-domino theory was prevalent because of three things—Chinese civil turmoil, lack of leadership in the Soviet Union, and their breaking of relations with each other. Do you know why the Korean war ended?" he asked.

I had to admit I was not sure.

"Three things contributed to its cessation: 1. The Death of Stalin, 2. A New President in the U.S. (Eisenhower) who had a mixed image of both a dove and a hawk, 3. The sick and tired feeling of Americans, along with the protests and political pressure from mothers of American Prisoners of War."

"In light of this," I queried, "what do you think could end the Vietnam war?"

"Possibly," he said, "the death of Mao Tse Tung, the installation of a new American leadership, and the growing unrest among people of the United States."

The Koreans, I explained, had contributed troops to the Vietnamese conflict. Why doesn't Japan send a token force?

He told me something I never realized.

Twenty years ago—after World War II, Japan adopted a Constitution in which Article 9 specifically prohibits Japan from entering into war as a means of resolving disagreements.

The Japanese, I was told, are indifferent to the war in Vietnam. I was not surprised, as I had found that this same indifference was prevalent in much of the United States.

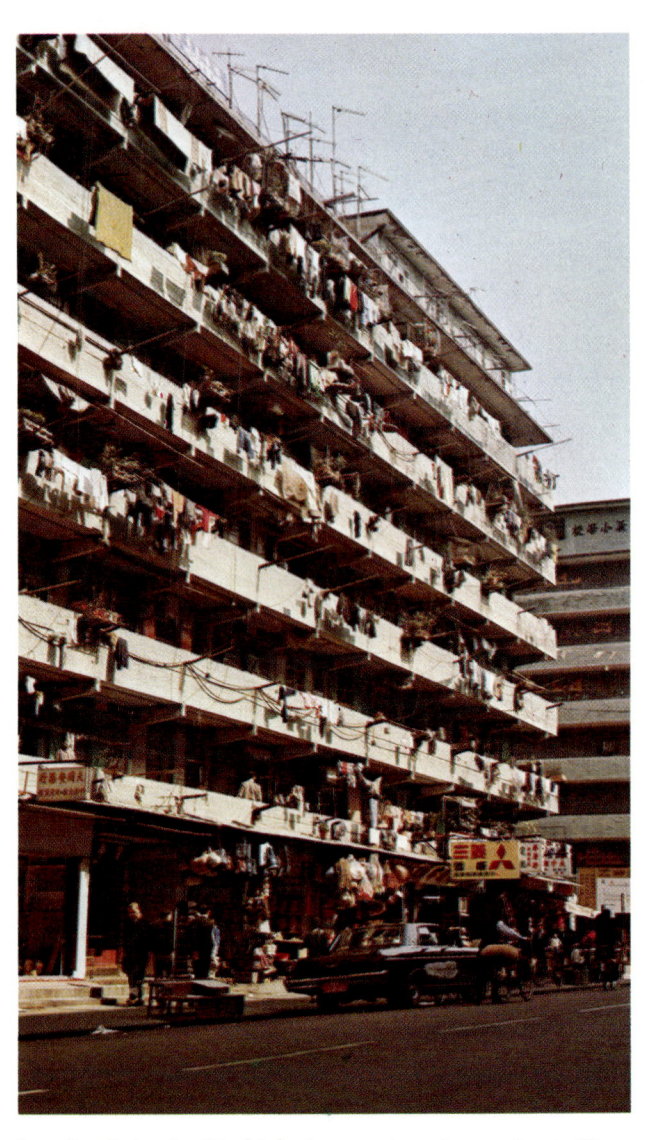

Imagine living in this high-rise apartment complex in Hong Kong where the humid heat reaches 115°, no elevators, and some 8-12 people live in one room!

HONG KONG
Royalty and Riot

While Queen Elizabeth was planting a tree at the Nautical College in Berkshire, England, and the American Woman's Association was holding a tea in Hong Kong—Hong Kong's teeming millions were sweltering under unbelievable living conditions that generated a riot leaving some 40 civilians and 7 policemen dead.

The day I arrived in Hong Kong the weather was hot and humid. The airport is in Kowloon—just across the bay from Hong Kong proper. It was in Kowloon that the July riots originated. The original disputes were two non-connected labor disputes.

One involved a Chinese-owned plastic factory in which the workers were demanding better working conditions and more pay. The other involved a dispute on the dismissal of a worker who alleged he had been struck by his European foreman.

Both started as peaceful demonstrations. But soon riots ensued and the communists moved in to take advantage of the fragile situation.

At Police Headquarters in Hong Kong I discussed the impact of the riots with a Chinese Police Officer (98% of Hong Kong is Chinese).

He related that in the last several weeks over 2500 people had been arrested—2000 of them in the Kowloon sector of Hong Kong. And after questioning about 600 were released —the others receiving sentences of from 3 months to 5 years.

Police restrictions were very tight. Anyone even spreading a rumor by word of mouth was subject to arrest.

The greatest number of casualties took place at the Chinese border—where Chinese Militiamen killed 5 Hong Kong police. The Chinese cut off their contract to supply water to Hong Kong.

Taiwan offered water free unconditionally—all the British had to do was send ships to get it. The British however took it under advisement.

I asked the Police Officer what steps the United Kingdom was taking to solve the social ills of Hong Kong.

He told me the Royal Government of Hong Kong had a 5 year plan—subject to review every 2 years. I asked for details of this plan. From his literature file he produced a richly printed 16 page booklet emblazoned with the United Kingdom Royal Crest.

The booklet, describing the plan to convert social ills, sells for $1 H.K.

Crumbs And Caviar

Back at the luxurious air-conditioned hotel I read this booklet. The introduction—describing what social progress other countries had adopted—took up one half of the space. The committee went on to explain that many of these solutions to social conditions were not applicable to Hong Kong. At some great length and at repeated intervals in the booklet, including the conclusion . . . the committee felt that voluntary organizations should shoulder much of the responsibility of Hong Kong's plight.

As I left the Hotel, British aristocracy were in full evening dress ready to attend a social function. The Indian doorman in full dress uniform and turban opened the door for me and I entered into a different world.

The frail beggar woman bent over with age asked for alms —"crumbs from the Master's table" and nearby even a dog was carrying a basket.

The hot humid air of Hong Kong brought me back to reality and in the crowded streets of an overpopulated city I wondered how a tree planting in England and a Ladies Tea in Hong Kong ever hoped to help a sick and starving populace.

"Subject to review in two years." Can the hungry wait that long? And how many more will die in this intermission simply because the ruling class doesn't want to dirty its hands with the root of the problems but rather subsist on the fruit of its vine?

A Desire for Wealth

I could not forget that it was the British who were responsible for importing opium into China about 1850.

Greedy to increase their trade, the British circumnavigated Chinese laws. The rulers of China had import restrictions on foreign trade and specifically prohibited the importation of opium from India. The Chinese destroyed many shipments of opium brought in by British merchants into the harbor of Canton.

The British East India Company used this action to attack several coastal cities in China. Revenues were falling and the British were anxious to increase this highly profitable trade. China stood no chance against the modern weaponry of England, and within two years five of her ports had opened to British trade.

Hong Kong was ceded to the British. Then the Chinese people were saturated with cheap and abundant supplies of opium. This served to enslave the natives and enriched the British exploiters of which Parliament had a direct financial interest.

Twelve years later China tried to throw off this yoke of drug bondage. A second Opium War ensued. China lost and the British again enlarged their trade in human suffering and death.

Today, as current as 1974, a British company...whose chairman is the former Lord Mayor of London...owns some 44,000 acres of land in Claiborne County, Tennessee. The land is leased to strip-mining companies that have left as a heritage black, poisoned waters that have killed wild life, ruined the mountains and left slag-heaps of shale along the once verdant countryside.

All for the sake of profit...but not for the miner, who many times ends up with black lung and is forced to end his days in poverty in a ramshackled house with no running water, no bathroom, sometimes no electricity, living along side a hole-pocked dirt road...surrounded by the putrefying stink from the mining refuse all about.

Even in today's world, the milk of human kindness is soured by the overwhelming desire for wealth by some.

When you start feeling sorry for yourself, keep this photograph in the back of your mind. Perhaps it will change your thoughts from self-pity to praise as you say "Thank you, Jesus...for dying for my sins, for bearing my burdens, for providing eternal life, for meeting my every need." I took this photograph in Hong Kong. I will never forget this scene. And it caused me to examine my life and to double my efforts in serving Christ.

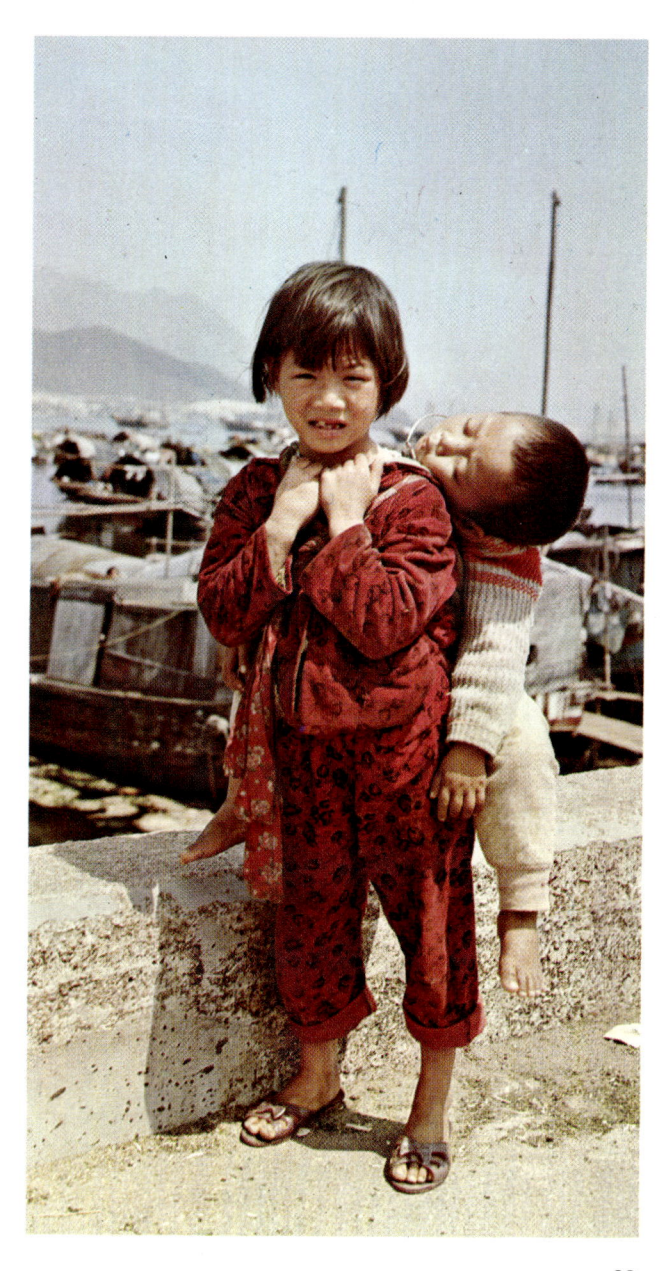

EDITORS:

WASHINGTON--THE WAR DEPARTMENT SAYS IT WILL ISSUE AN ANNOUNCEMENT AROUND 5 A.M. NO INDICATION HAS BEEN GIVEN OF ITS NATURE.

THE A.P.

FLASH   WASHINGTON--ARMY ANNOUNCES ROME BOMBED

BULLETIN   1ST LEAD INVASION

BY REYNOLDS PACKARD   UNITED PRESS STAFF CORRESPONDENT

ALLIED HEADQUARTERS, NORTH AFRICA, SEPT. 3.--(UP)--ALLIED FORCES UNDER GEN. DWIGHT D. EISENHOWER OPENED THE LONG-HERALDED SECOND FRONT IN EUROPE EARLY TODAY, STRIKING BY LAND, SEA AND AIR AGAINST THE BOMB-SHATTERED SOUTHERN TIP OF THE ITALIAN MAINLAND.

TODAY IS B-DAY--6

The Evening Bulletin

FINAL

PHILADELPHIA, TUESDAY, MAY 8, 1945   THREE CENTS

V-E Day Proclaimed

Truman Announces ...unday will be ... of Prayer

WESTERN UNION

CLASS OF SERVICE

This is a full-rate Telegram or Cablegram unless its deferred character is indicated by a suitable symbol above or preceding the address.

A. N. WILLIAMS, PRESIDENT

NLT = Cable Night Letter
Ship Radiogram

The filing time shown in the date line on telegrams and day letters is STANDARD TIME at point of origin. Time of receipt is STANDARD TIME at point of destination

PT185   NL PD= SANFRANCISCO CALIF DEC 22

MISS MARY STEVENSON=

4346 NORTH 8 ST=

ARRIVED IN SANFRANCISCO DEC 21 MERRY CHRISTMAS DARLING=

SALEM.

AT SAN FRANCISCO

Miscellaneous personnel on following: Monterey from Manila, 4,347; Hunter Liggett from Guam, 2,371; Attu from Leyte, 1,311; Zaurak from Shanghai, 1,019 Navy; Copahee from Pearl Harbor, 527 Navy; Circe from Japan, 479 Navy; Wantuck from Pearl Harbor, 130 Navy; Polana from Guam, 103 Navy; Plunkett from Adak, 165 Navy; LST 168 from Pearl Harbor, 106 Navy; also few each on Lightning, LST 613, Belazon Smith, John Sedgwick, LST 762, Cinnamon, Torchwood, Silver Bell and Melucta.

21.

THE COMPANY WILL APPRECIATE SUGGESTIONS FROM ITS PATRONS CONCERNING ITS SERVICE

CONFUSION, MISUNDERSTANDING AND LIES

It was Sunday evening, July 23. The sleek personal jet of General Westmoreland has just landed at Tan San Nuit Air Base outside of Saigon.

And with the news and wire services . . . I was there . . . in the VIP lounge with cameras and tape recorder. For the first time I would witness a press interview and it was to be most revealing.

One reporter asked: "Sir, there continues to be some confusion about the infiltration rate. In Washington they say that only about 1000 North Vietnamese a month come down to South Vietnam. In Saigon, your command says about 8000."

"Well, there is a time lag from the time infiltration occurs and our knowledge of this" . . . commented Westmoreland.

"General, what do you consider the problem with the South Vietnamese Army and how long do you think it will take for them to become an effective fighting force?" queried a reporter.

"Well, I think the South Vietnamese army has made great progress during the 3 1/2 years that I've been associated with them. I think the record speaks for itself," Westmoreland replied.

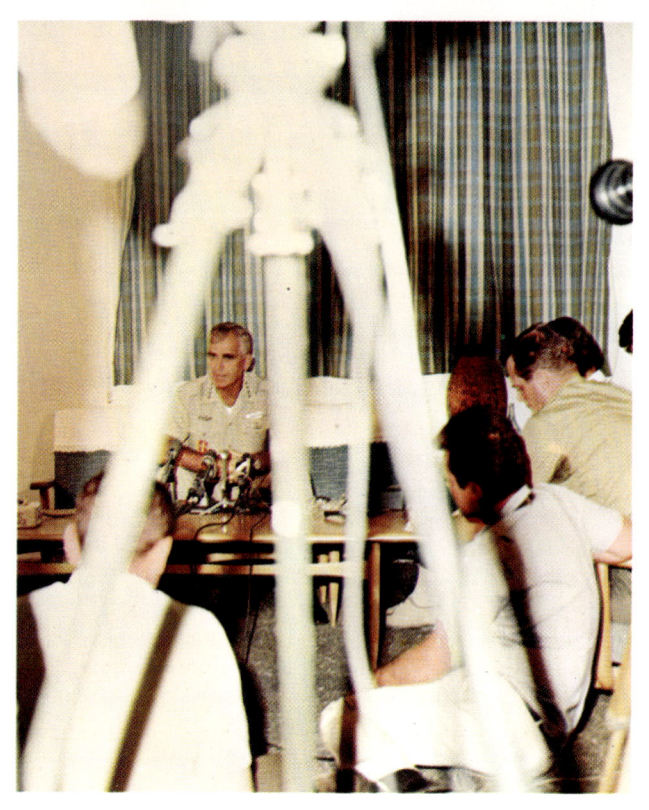

Press conference with General Westmoreland at airport in Vietnam in August, 1967.

"General, do you feel there is a stalemate now in the war?"

"Well, I don't accept the statement. We've made steady progress during the last 2 years."

"Can you outline some of the progress you've made in the last 6 months?"

"Well, ah, areas that are now secured, roads that are open, canals that are now in daily use, population has been brought under control, VC base areas that have been invaded and destroyed, ah, the initiative has shifted in the past 2 years," . . . replied Westmoreland.

"Do you consider areas secure when we can move our troops out of there?"

"Well," replied Westmoreland, "I think security is a relative thing. If our troops were moved out, I think without question the Viet Cong would move back in. This is the nature of the conflict.

Our ground strategy in the South must be defensive . . . because we must protect the South Vietnamese from aggression and give them a freedom of choice."

This is what the public would hear over their mass news media. This is what they want to hear . . . and it would be dished out in the fine, cloaked language of the big brass.

But what about the man in the field—the GI daily meeting the VC head-on? What about the officers meeting problems and being frustrated because of the enormity of the impossible job—being run 10,000 miles away and, as the Indians say, "with a forked tongue?"

Security And Death

Two days later I was out in the field . . . . . I talked with these men, asking them specific questions answered previously in glowing terms by General Westmoreland.

I found a completely different story.

"Are the roads secure?"

They laughed in my face. Everyone I interviewed said basically the same thing. "NO ROAD IN VIETNAM IS SECURE. We're always subject to sniper fire and people are getting killed."

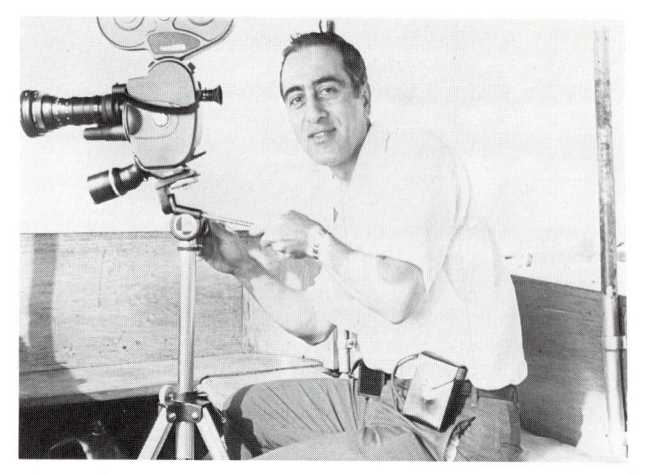

The Author taking motion pictures of floating market in Bangkok, Thailand.

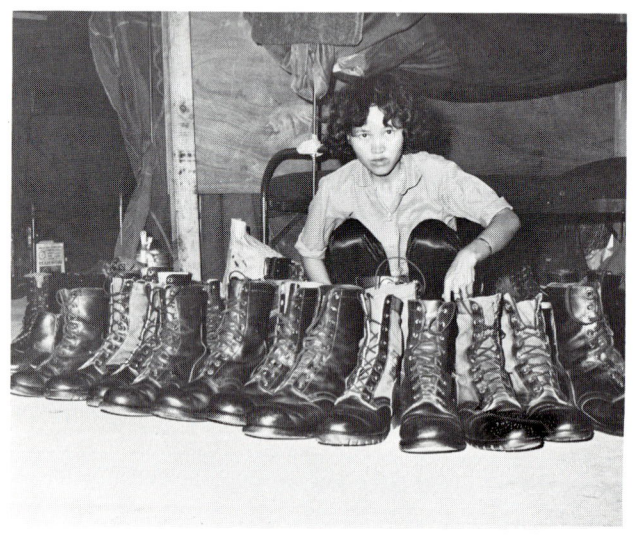

Thousands of Vietnamese were employed on U.S. bases. High level officers were constantly concerned about the ensuing inflationary economy.

Even around the perimeter of Saigon I interviewed those who had been wounded in that area in fresh battles from so-called secure areas.

"What about the great progress the South Vietnamese Army has made?"

> "What progress" they replied. "They're not pulling their own weight. Why, there's 500,000 kids roaming the streets that should be in uniform. But they don't want that because then the United States would pull out and their economy of leeching America would suffer."

I was to see many examples of how the Vietnamese people bleed Americans blind. A familiar sign in Vietnam is a small decal showing a pair of clasped hands. It signifies the Hands over the Ocean, ideas of the Good White Father United States benevolently supplying free aid to alleviate the suffering of other countries.

What happened to these goods when they came over? Here are a few examples I learned first hand.

> An Air Force base finds it needs a water pump. In the States, such a pump would cost about $50. They are authorized to go into the city and purchase this pump from the Vietnamese. On the pump, the bright Clasped Hands decal is evident—a free gift from Uncle Sam to the Vietnamese people. Our Air Force must buy the pump . . . and at the dollar exchange rate—at $250.00. So the Vietnamese get a double bonus, a FREE GIFT and 100% profit at over 4 times the value of the pump.

Such scruples are not reserved only for Americans. They bleed their own people, too.

> An example—another clasped-hands project: Similac —a powdered food basic for babies. Given by the U.S. Government to be distributed free to the Vietnamese people. Cost about $1.25 a can in the U.S. A South Vietnamese woman excitedly shows a G.I. what she has bought—a can of Similac. What did you pay for it? $1.50," she replied.

> Cheated this time by her own countrymen.

A pilot, authorized to secure sun glasses from Army Supply free because they are a must for flying . . . finds they are

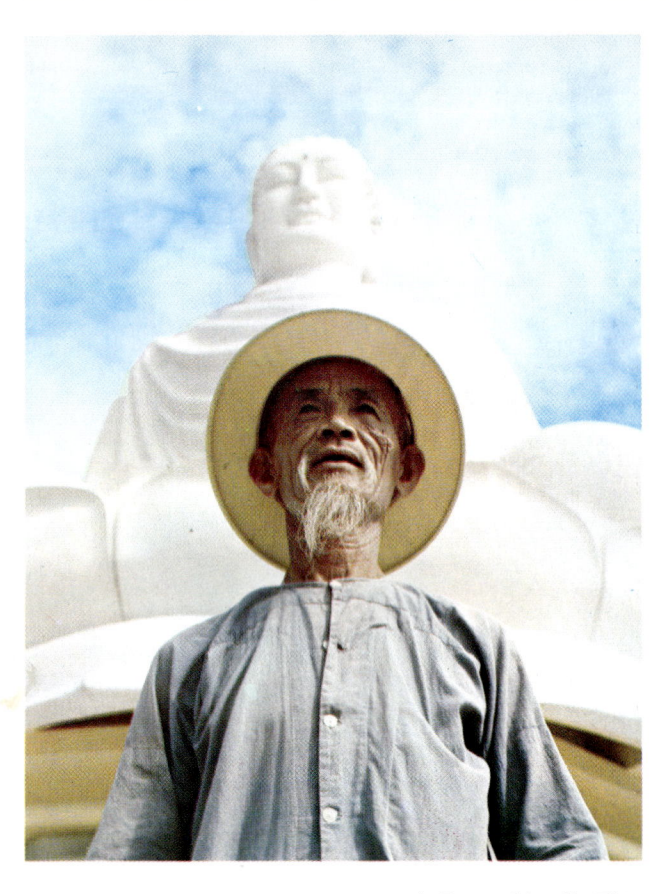

Friend or foe? Not even a seasoned GI could tell. This Vietnamese could be friend during the day and foe at night.

unavailable at supply. He walks down the street and these same regulation glasses are displayed by sidewalk vendors.

A Refined Graft

In other wars graft and bribes were born . . . and they were even nurtured in Washington, D.C., but one thing you must give the Vietnamese credit for, they have not only quickly learned but very skillfully refined the art of wholesale graft and open bribe . . . starting from the top echelon all the way down.

The GI's I talked with—officers and enlisted men alike— who have had daily contact both with the Vietnamese Army and the people came back with the same impressions.

> The Vietnamese Army is lazy, indifferent (with a few exceptions) and are more than willing to let Americans bear the brunt of the war. The Vietnamese people have no sense of loyalty and couldn't care less about who won the war. Their main concern is that we will pull out and they will lose their gold mine of leeching Americans.

It would be presumptuous on my part, spending only 10 days in Vietnam, to make brash statements of my findings. My own findings were, however, after in the field interviews—substantiated by those who were in positions to know and make authoritative comments.

One such avenue I approached was to interview leading news correspondents and photographers who had witnessed battles and covered all of South Vietnam during long areas of time on the field.

The consensus of their remarks was that the South Vietnamese are indolent and could care less about the war. They have a lack of loyalty and unity, and some will take every opportunity to rob you.

The War That Never Ends

They cherish a war of attrition. And America—regardless of what people read back home—can never secure Vietnam—unless they man for man, post soldiers in every nook and cranny every hour of every day forever . . . and if they do this, they should always keep one hand on their back pocket—to secure their wallet.

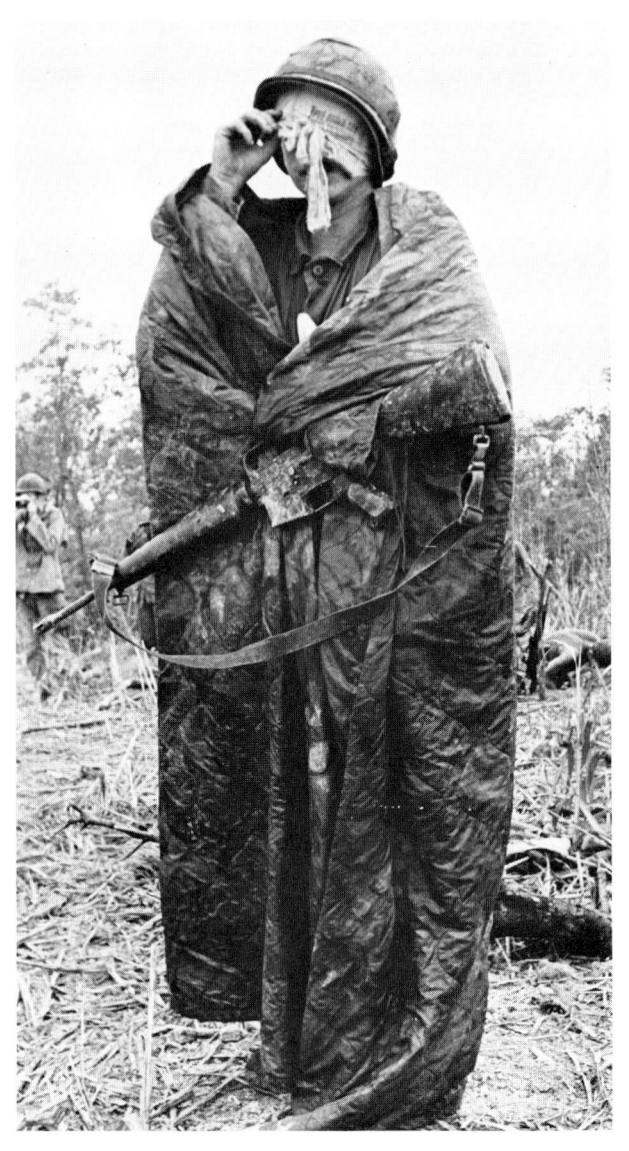

This photograph etches the hopelessness and the futility of war. Photo was taken in Vietnam.

In fairness to the Vietnamese I must admit I met some very nice people, but these were the very poor, down trodden unfortunates humbled by the conditions of poverty in which they live.

Strange Economics

It was an odd war when we had to pay the Vietnam government rent for using their land, then send them Hands Across the Ocean Free food and supplies, only to have to buy it back again at high, inflated prices. It's a well known fact that vegetables trucked into U.S. bases from inland had to pay VC tax along the way, sometimes taxed 5 or 10 times before the truck reached the Army base. Tomatoes which should be selling for about 20¢ a pound finally arrived at U.S. bases at 60¢ a pound. So in effect we not only pay the Vietnamese but through the tax structure helped support the military arm of the VC who in turn used the U.S. money to buy guns and ammunition to kill our young American boys in the prime of their life.

Newspapers the world over carried Secretary of Defense McNamara's statement that some part of Westmoreland's forces were not being used efficiently and that more troops should be taken from support units and put up into front line units.

When asked this question by newsmen at that airport interview, General Westmoreland replied: "I don't think Secretary McNamara made that statement—at least he has not discussed this with me. I don't believe his remarks were intended to apply to elements in my commands."

Confusion and misunderstanding appeared to have full sway here. Then, too, newsmen who wrote too realistic a story reporting the facts on Vietnam, in some instances had their articles sent back by their newspaper with the comment to rewrite in a more conciliatory fashion.

When will American leaders be honest with its people? How much longer must we fight entangling wars, and support the enemy through the morass of corruption and graft?

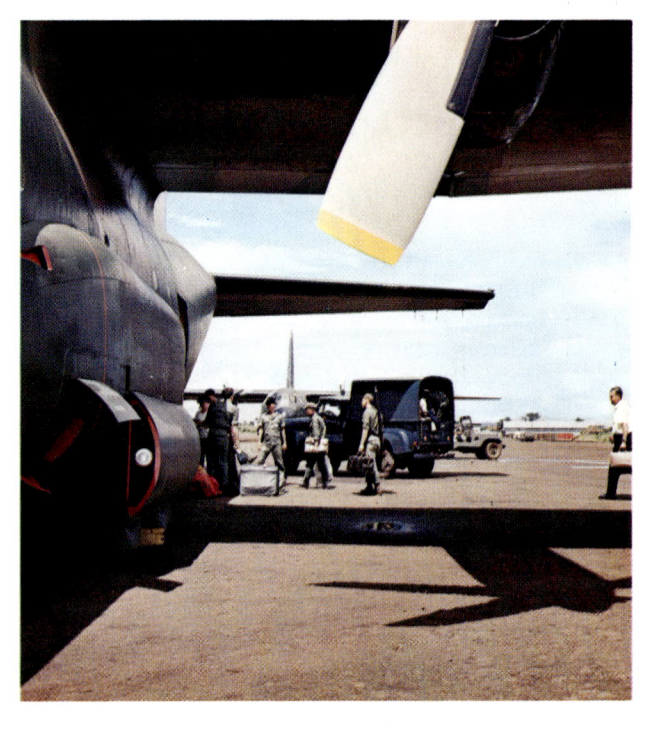

Accompanying returning servicemen, our troop plane landed briefly at Pleiku air base.

VIETNAM AT LAST!

Leaving Japan, the main purpose of my mission was soon to be fulfilled . . . meeting my son.

Our plane stopped briefly in Hong Kong and with a day's layover I visited the city of riots. It was but a brief introduction for what I was to see in Vietnam.

Flying over Vietnam all the passengers were looking out the window for some signs of war. But all we could see were the verdant mountains and mist covered valleys. It was hard to imagine that down below men were battling for their lives.

And the reality of war did not become evident until we landed at the Saigon airport.

Accustomed to fancy air terminals and efficient service, the Saigon airport was to be quite a shocking contrast.

The terminal looked like a ramshackled, overgrown barn ringed by Vietnamese soldiers and military aircraft. We were hustled off the plane and herded into a small room. And then utter confusion began. Little Vietnamese men scurrying back and forth shouting unintelligible instructions in a language foreign to us . . . black pajamaed women trying to quiet bawling babies. People shoving and waiting and waiting. And the smells and sweat of Vietnam became very evident.

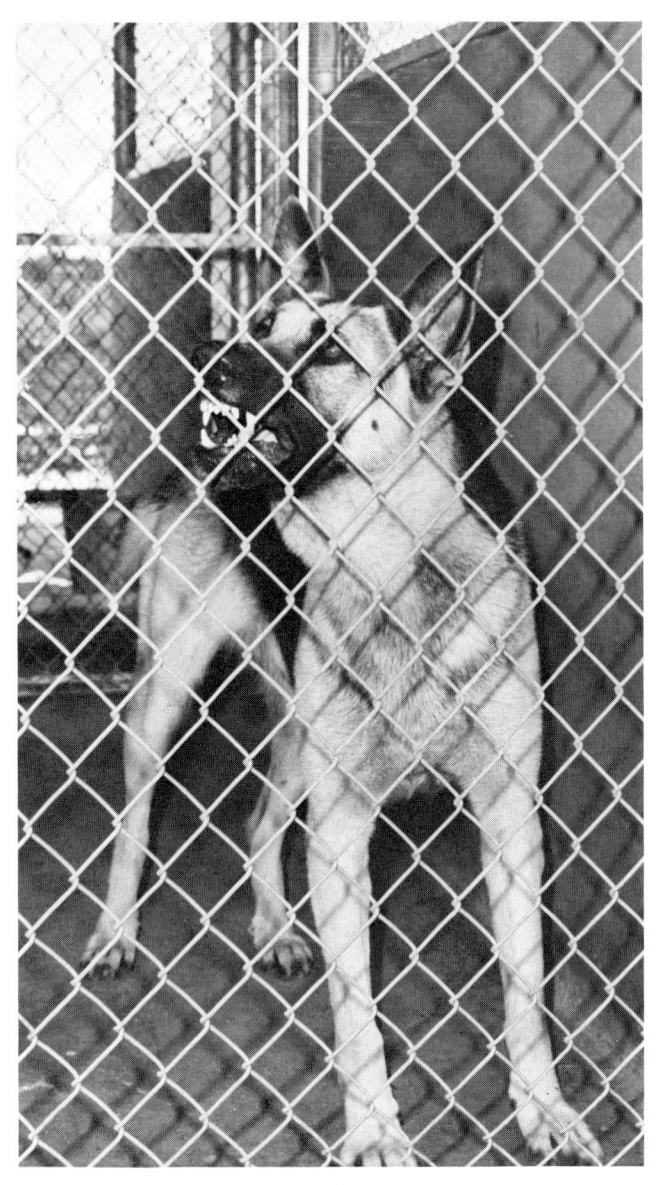

With all the sophistication of modern warfare, the sentry dog still plays a vital role against sneak attacks.

After finally passing through customs I tried to get a cab. Cabs were not allowed within the secure perimeter of the airport. A few "cleared" cars provide transportation. No markings, no meters, these broken down cars become Saigon's deluxe mode of transportation. My hotel was some 20 minutes away.

I was anxious to see my son and tired of waiting. With my film equipment my bags weighed over 100 pounds—not a comfortable load to carry in the oppresive humid air of Vietnam.

The driver sloshed through the mud and put my bags in the car. While these drivers spoke little English they do understand U.S. currency. My driver wanted $7 to drive me to my hotel. By this time I had exhausted my patience— got out of the car and told him to take out my bags—all 100 pounds. The trip was worth only $2. "I'm not interested in buying your country," I told him, "I just want to get to my hotel!"

I finally got to the hotel by way of another cab driver for only $3. It was a French hotel—the Embassy. My room rate was $20 a day. It was worth about $4 a day.

Corruption And Inflation

I had just received my first taste of war—corruption and inflation. And driving through the streets, I saw the filth, mountains of trash littering the curbs, women and children huddled in the mud eating their lunch cooked on outdoor stoves—surrounded by dirt and flies while barebottom tots were using the streets as their bathroom.

The traffic of Saigon is like a Mack Sennett movie. Literally thousands of motorcycles and pedi-cycles flood the inadequate narrow streets. Red traffic lights are a luxury Saigon doesn't enjoy except at three or four main intersections. Everyone for himself seems to be the order of the day.

This was war. Barbed wire compounds, sentry gates manned by Vietnam and U.S. soldiers with arms drawn . . . the overpopulated city seemed to accept war simply as the normal way of life.

Suddenly I Was Lonely

Finally reaching my hotel room, I showered and rested. It

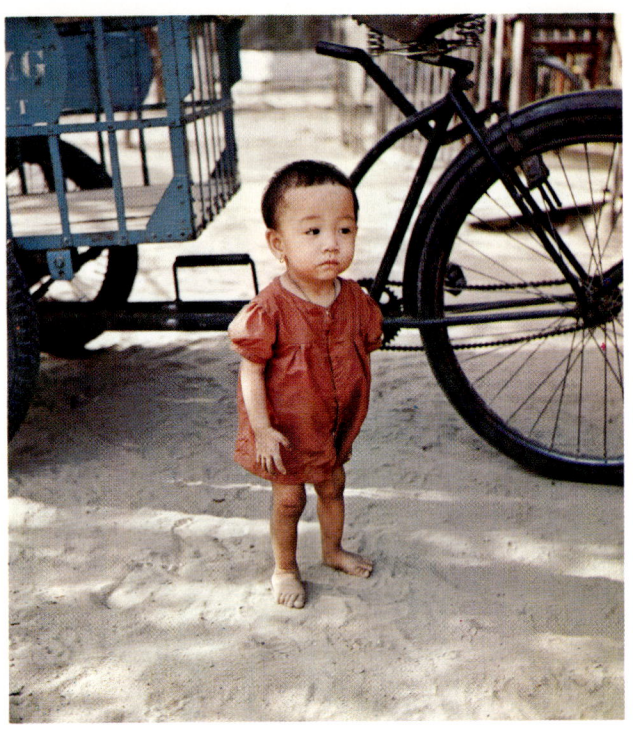

Photo by Dennis Kirban

This tiny waif wanders aimlessly in the sand of Nha Trang, bewildered by the noise of war.

was hard to believe. Here I was in Vietnam. Soon I would be seeing my son. Outside it was drizzling and at long last a weary homesickness was creeping in. I missed home—my wife, my children, my loved ones. I knew I was entering a hazardous area that could take my life (as it did three other reporters). I did not have to be in Vietnam. Right now I could be sitting in an easy chair at home in air-conditioned comfort watching TV and sipping a Coke. Instead I was perspiring in a lonely hotel room 10,000 miles from home in a strange city in a land at war . . . a war that could erupt into personal tragedy with the next step or by the ever grinning Vietnamese bellboy who held his hand out for a tip.

And this made that night even more lonely. I had chosen this course—because while I longed for my family I was also concerned for my son.

And torn betwixt two poles I felt duty-bound to do my best to fathom the reasons for war and contribute my small part in achieving peace. The stakes were high—my son's life and that of thousands of other sons.

If tragedy should befall my son I could never forgive myself for not having at least actively tried to resolve some of the war's issues—and seeing him once again.

Sure I was homesick. But mine was a small sacrifice—theirs was not. That night my prayers were moistened with tears and tomorrow would bring me closer to a grand reunion with Dennis.

It would be two days before I could see my son—two days of endless red tape securing the necessary correspondent's accreditation cards.

I had to secure these "passports to Vietnam" from both the Vietnamese and U.S. government offices in Saigon. These cards are highly valued as they give you free access to the entire country—free plane transportation and permission to eat in officer's mess and stay in officer's quarters.

Dennis...This Is Your Dad

At the bank where I had my U.S. dollars converted into Vietnamese currency the teller, a young Vietnamese, cautioned me to stay away from crowds and particularly groups of children who had been trained to be adept pickpockets.

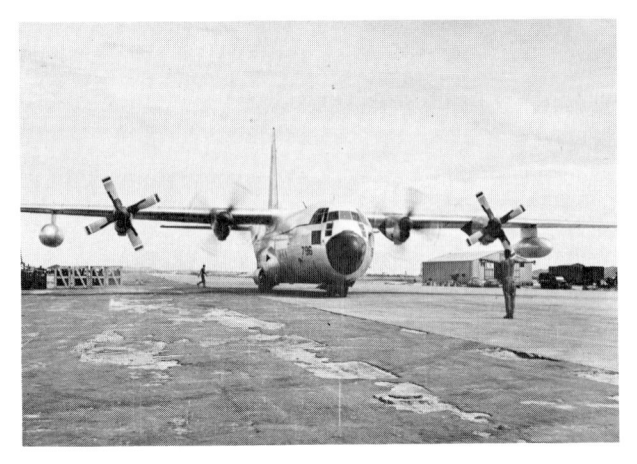

A lumbering C-130 lands at Tan San Nuit.

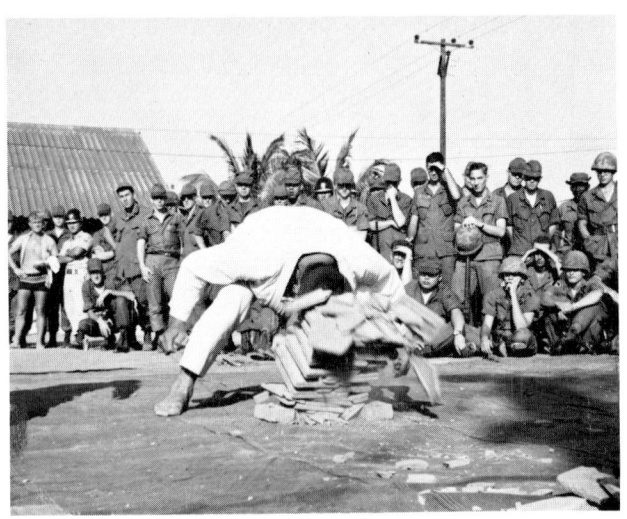

Photo by Dennis Kirban

A Korean soldier demonstrates the power of karate by breaking a pile of bricks with his head!

Used to the luxury of the American telephone system I decided to call my son from Press Headquarters in Saigon. I found this next to impossible. On my second day my phone call reached his headquarters office. Coincidentally, he was on duty at the time.

One can't imagine the thrill I had when on the other end of the phone I heard: "Headquarters office, Pvt. Dennis Kirban speaking sir."

I paused a moment and then said, "Dennis, this is your dad."

The next few minutes were filled with excited conversation as father and son had a wonderful reunion via phone. The next day I was able to get on one of the regular Army flights to Nha Trang where Dennis was stationed.

At the Tan San Nuit airport I boarded a lumbering C-130 Army transport plane. With me were about 50 soldiers—most of them shouldering duffel bags and rifles. No comfortable seats here—just 4 rows of nylon strapping running the full length of the plane. Almost windowless, one flies in semi-darkness the entire trip.

Flying direct to Nha Trang would be only one hour. But this particular flight took four hours. It was a milk run flight with Nha Trang the last stop.

At Pleiku most of the soldiers left the plane—lined up in formation and went marching to their new assignment where fighting was clearly evidenced around the perimeter of the air strip. Hastily pushed off the air strip so we could land was a destroyed fighter plane.

The pilot invited me into the cockpit and as we rose above Pleiku he pointed out recently made bomb craters and the defoliated mountain ranges.

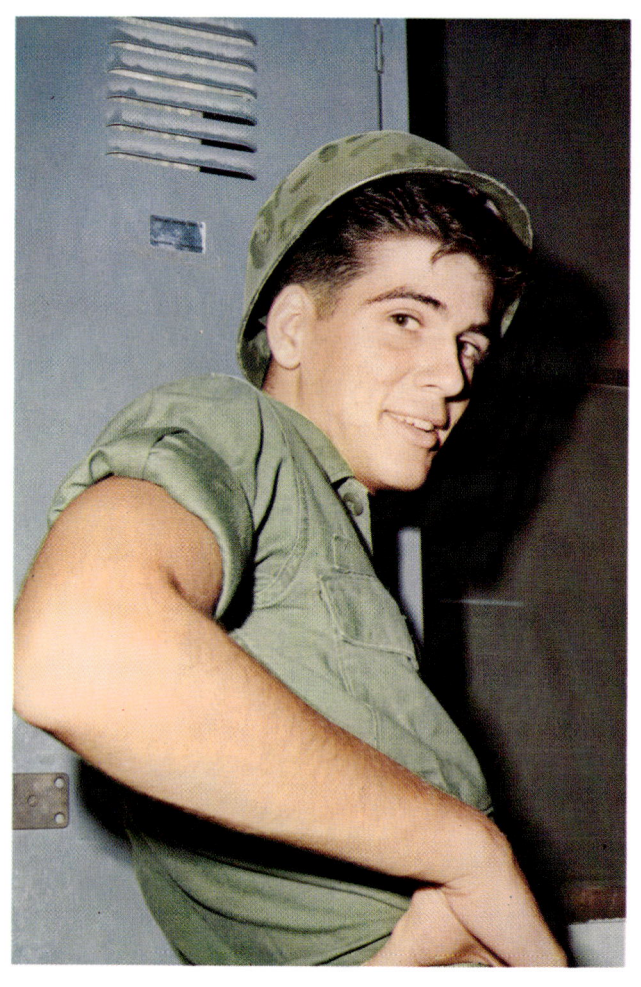

Dennis Kirban in Vietnam.

THE GRAND REUNION

What would it be like when I first met my son, Dennis, I reflected? This was no ordinary trip. Our family had deep religious roots. With so much emphasis on body counts in this war, my wife and I often talked about whether our son could even kill another man. We hoped this set of circumstances would never arise.

A Mother's Advice

"Shoot to wound—but not to kill" my wife once wrote Dennis. Dennis was not the belligerent, hard hearted boy. As a youngster he always kept a pet toad or frog in the window well . . . and he would often come home with a puppy or a kitten that needed love and nourishment. One day he found a raccoon near the highway. He brought it home. He carefully watched over a brood of white mice one year, rabbits another. He loved to build—first H. O. trains—then cars. He hated inefficiency and loved to keep things in perfect order. And most of all he loved his individual freedom.

One day at Fort Huachuca a drunken soldier came in the barracks—for no reason at all—yanked him out of bed and started hitting him. Dennis stepped back and did not provoke the fight further. Results—a cut head with stitches and KP because the C.O. thought he started it.

I'll never forget the day I visited him at basic training camp at Fort Gordon, Georgia. I was picking him and some buddies up for their Christmas leave.

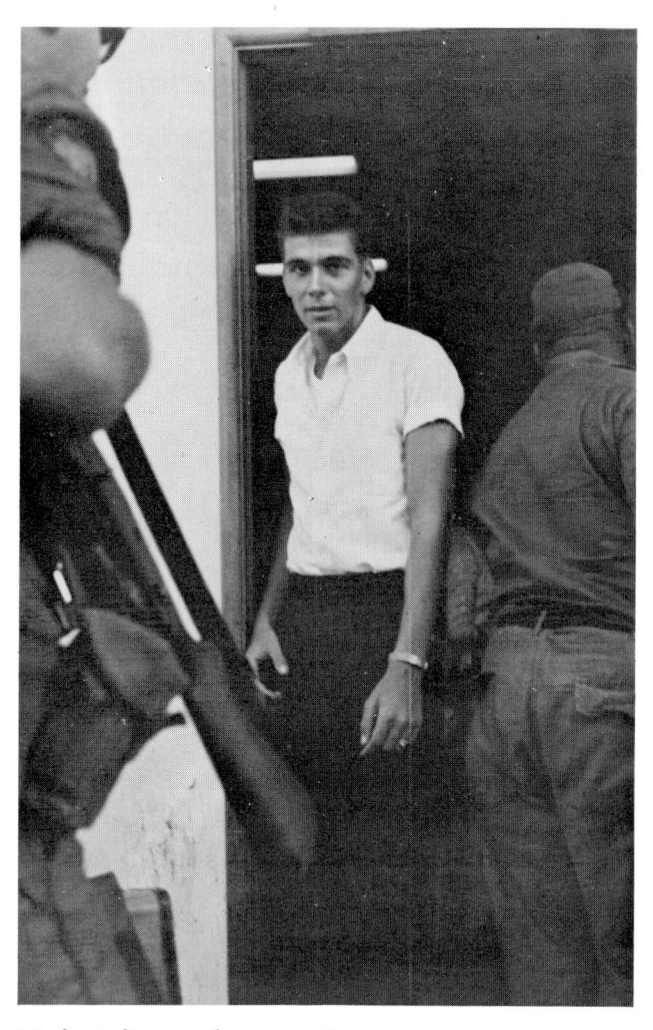

My first glimpse of my son, Dennis, as I got off the C130 at Nha Trang, Vietnam. It was a day I will never forget.

Where Does Duty End

As I entered the barracks I heard a continual barrage of the most colorful obscene cursing I had ever experienced. What was happening, I wondered, as I walked to the end of the barracks. I soon found out it was the sergeant instructing the G.I.'s in the moving of some new cots and bags into the barracks. The more I looked at him in disgust the bluer his language became. I told Dennis later that perhaps the best present for the sergeant would be a Webster dictionary . . . so he could discover some more acceptable words in the English language.

Another incident occurred on the remote area of his base in the supply depot. From time to time there has been skirmishes here with Viet Cong infiltration and a guard killed. Dennis was concerned about pulling guard duty in this lonely outpost. His turn came and his guard was in the early hours of the morning. After it was over he wondered what in the world he was guarding that was placing his life in jeopardy.

It was a warehouse of beer.

"Suppose," he wrote, "I had been killed at this post guarding a warehouse of beer . . . and I don't even drink!"

He enlisted in the Army for three years believing he would receive better schooling. But when he saw that draftees received the same opportunities as he—but with only two years to serve—he was disappointed.

Giving up three years of his life in a "mark time" program he wistfully looked forward to his day of "freedom." Neither he nor we believed in the necessity of this war and the more we saw of it the greater our convictions became.

On the plus side, the Army training quickly matured him—gave him a responsible set of values and for the first time in his life was able to appreciate what many of us, when we are young, take for granted.

My Son! My Son!

The long plane ride was over and our C-130 pulled up to the ramp at the Nha Trang airport. I was half-way around the world and my mission was soon to be completed. Would I recognize my son? Had the war affected him in any way? I knew one thing, it would be a wonderful reunion but it

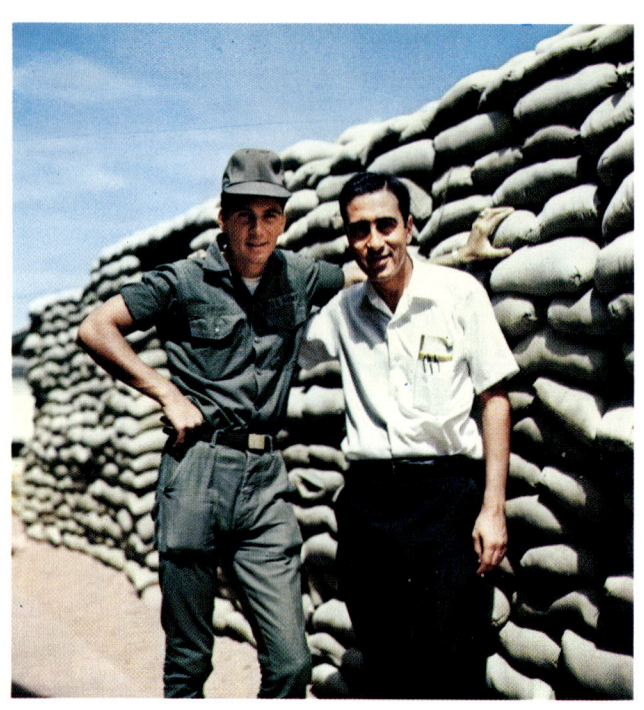

The grand reunion...Dennis with Dad.

would retie home bands and parting would be so much more difficult.

It seemed like an eternity before the propellers stopped turning and the doors swung open. Only the baggage handlers were at planeside so I walked towards the low terminal building carrying my camera bag with my camera around my neck. I wanted to get a picture of his face as he first spotted me. There were many doors—which one was the right one to enter?

From one doorway at the terminal I heard a happy shout, "Hey, Dad, over here!"

There was no mistake. It was my son's voice. I snapped the photo as he came running out to shake my hand.

It was a reunion neither of us will ever forget. Dressed in civvies he was no longer the thin, lanky, pale kid I had remembered. He had a deep tan and bulging, rippling muscles, which I later learned were as a result of a weight-lifting program he practiced in his spare time in Vietnam.

He excitedly told me about his weight-lifting accomplishments and I gladly let him handle my 100-pound suitcase and camera bag.

He was proud of his dad and everyone at the airport looked at us in awe. Even the Colonel had loaned us a jeep and my son received 5 days duty-free.

The red carpet was out.

> "To think," the guys were saying, "that your father would fly all the way over here to see you!"

It made quite an impression on the base and there was no doubt in my mind that this experience alone made the trip worthwhile.

This was the first opportunity he had to get behind a wheel in months and driving the jeep into Nha Trang Dennis relished every minute of it.

That night we had a steak dinner in the best restaurant in town with shrimp cocktail and all the trimmings. I brought him up to date on the news back home and we reminisced about the good old days.

When we got back to the barracks I decided to bunk in an

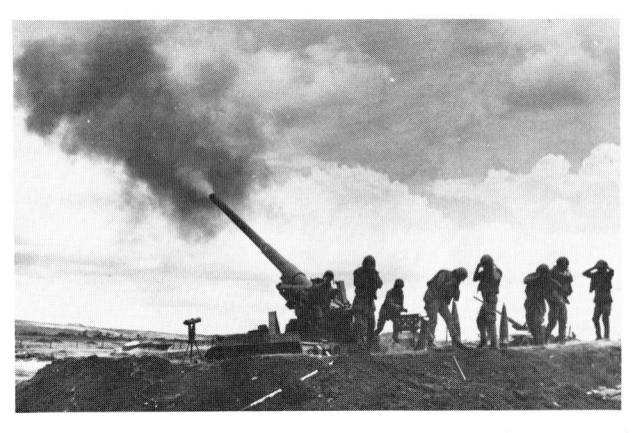

American soldiers brace themselves against the noise of the 175mm self-propelled gun as they fire from their fire support base at Mai Loc, south of the DMZ in South Vietnam.

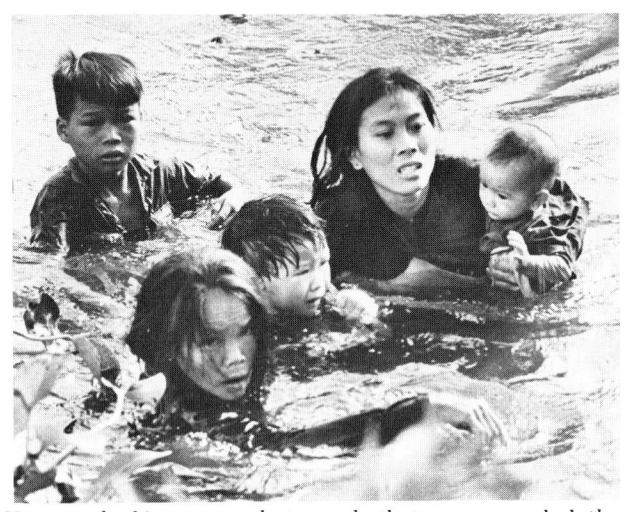

You are looking at a photograph that was awarded the Pulitzer Prize for News Photography in 1966. It depicts a Vietnamese mother and her children wading a river to escape an attack on their village.

empty bed a couple feet from my son. While I could have stayed in officer's quarters and ate in officer's mess, I wanted to be an ordinary G.I. again—just like my son.

That night together we went to the enlisted men's club, had soft drinks and hot dogs and continued our happy reunion.

Many in the group wondered who I was—some thought I was Dennis' brother. It isn't everyday that a civilian drops in and spends a week following an enlisted man's routine and sleeping at night in his barracks.

Late that night we went to bed in a state of happiness and yet with homesick dreams of loved ones back in the States.

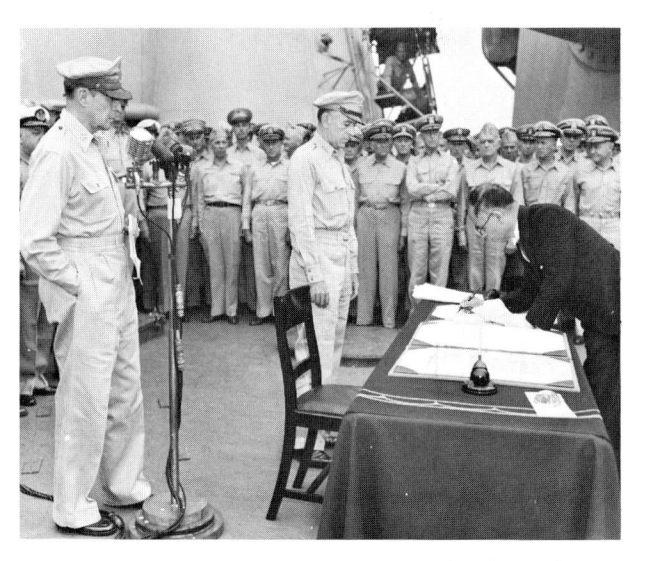

I fought in World War 2 and I remember the thrill of standing aboard an AKA cargo-troop transport en route to Tokyo. Suddenly on that bright sunny day I saw sailors on other ships tossing their white hats high in the air...the war was over! Peace had finally come!

Here, General MacArthur watches as the foreign minister Manoro Shigemitsu of Japan signs the surrender document on the USS Missouri, September 2, 1945. Little did I realize, that some 22 years later, my son would be fighting...again, in Asia!

65

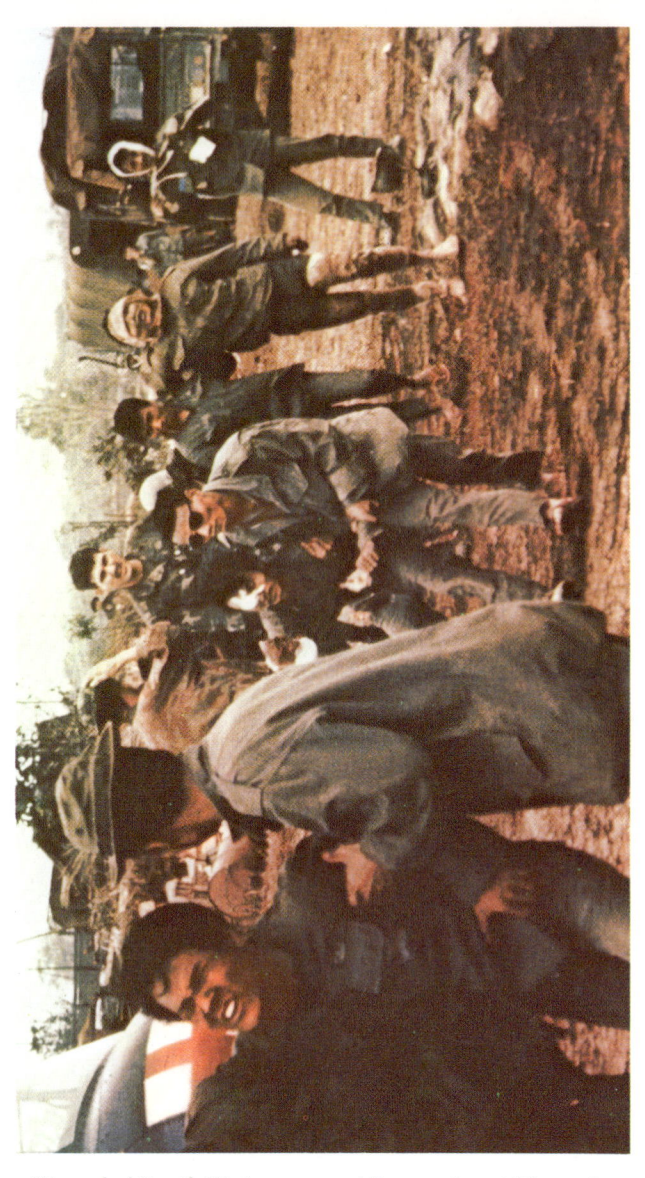

Wounded South Vietnamese soldiers arrive at Khesanh medical evacuation station for treatment.

THE GLORY IS FOR THE LIVING

At the daily 5 PM briefing to newsmen, casualties were described as "light" . . . 36 Americans killed in sporadic action.

It was just a statistic.

Then I witnessed the reality of that statistic.

And for the first time . . . I wept.

Tan San Nuit—an odd sounding name—is the headquarters of one of the largest Air Force Bases in Vietnam, located in Saigon.

This sprawling complex clearly defines the military might of the United States. It is bustling with activity.

My tour of the base began with the Medical Transfer Hospital. I watched as both stretcher and ambulatory casualties were loaded on to air-conditioned buses to be transferred to waiting airplanes that would whisk them to Japan, Hawaii or the United States for further treatment.

Those whose wounds were not too critical would be returned to the field to again face enemy fire and possible death.

Little did they realize that just on the other side of the wall lay their fallen comrades who didn't make it.

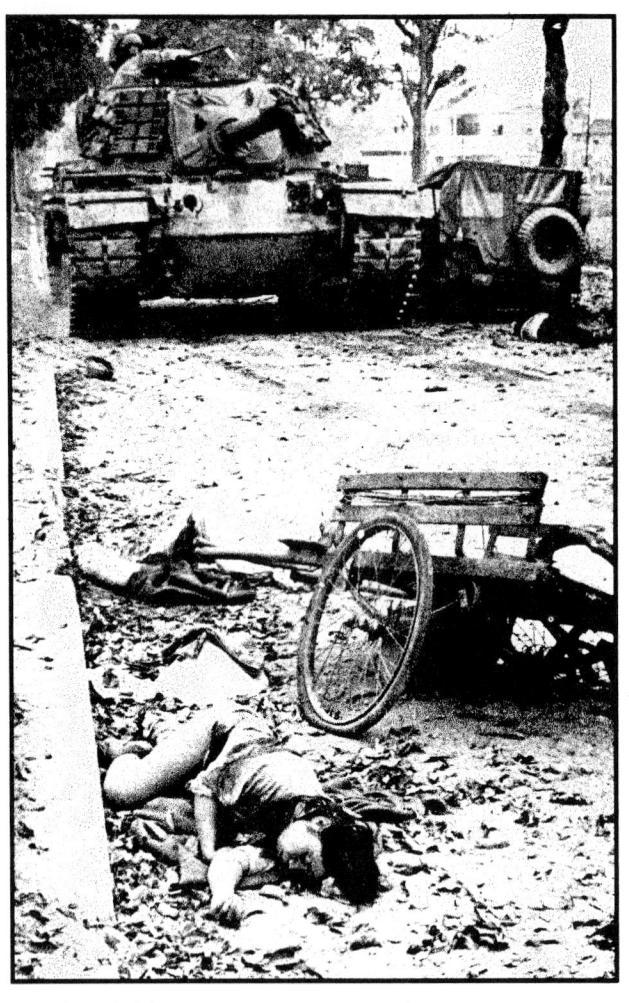

For this child, peace is a cemetery plot in Vietnam.

I interviewed several on the one bus I accompanied to planeside. They were bound for Japan, a sorespot in the eyes of many Japanese who do not want to become involved in the war.

One soldier, hit by shrapnel, had lain 1 1/2 hours in the field, afraid to move. A VC kicked him and he feigned death. The battle continued for 3 hours leaving 18 in his group wounded and 3 killed. Within 4 hours he was in a Field Hospital receiving treatment. Now he was destined for Japan for 2 more months of convalescent care.

All this occurred just 40 or 50 miles outside of Saigon on a so called "secure" road.

The Viet Cong are known for their atrocites, but the Vietnamese contributes its share too. In fact, even U.S. servicemen, embittered by the war, seeing their buddies killed, understandably develop a kill instinct that permits them to kill women and children if they feel that there are sympathetic or hostile VC in the area.

This fact was brought home to me by airmen who would rather kill first and ask questions afterward.

It's one of the bitter realities that war brings.

War's Greatest Tragedy

On the ready-room wall, where wounded are prepared for transfer, is posted a sign—"Tell God that you love him." But I noticed an embarrassing silence as the stretchers were being prepared.

There was no glory here—no tremendous thrill. One soldier I talked to just thanked God he was at least alive because some of his buddies didn't make it.

"How are the dead treated?" I asked the Information Officer at the Air Base. I soon found the word "dead" is not used. They are referred to as "remains." Later I was to be told by the Colonel in charge of Mortuary that many times there are very little remains.

For those who have paid the supreme sacrifice I was sure some dedicated ceremony would be conducted at planeside. I was told that in the beginning of the war such was the case. A detachment of men would stand at attention and a brief ceremony would ensue.

But the rising casualty rate and increasing outshipment of

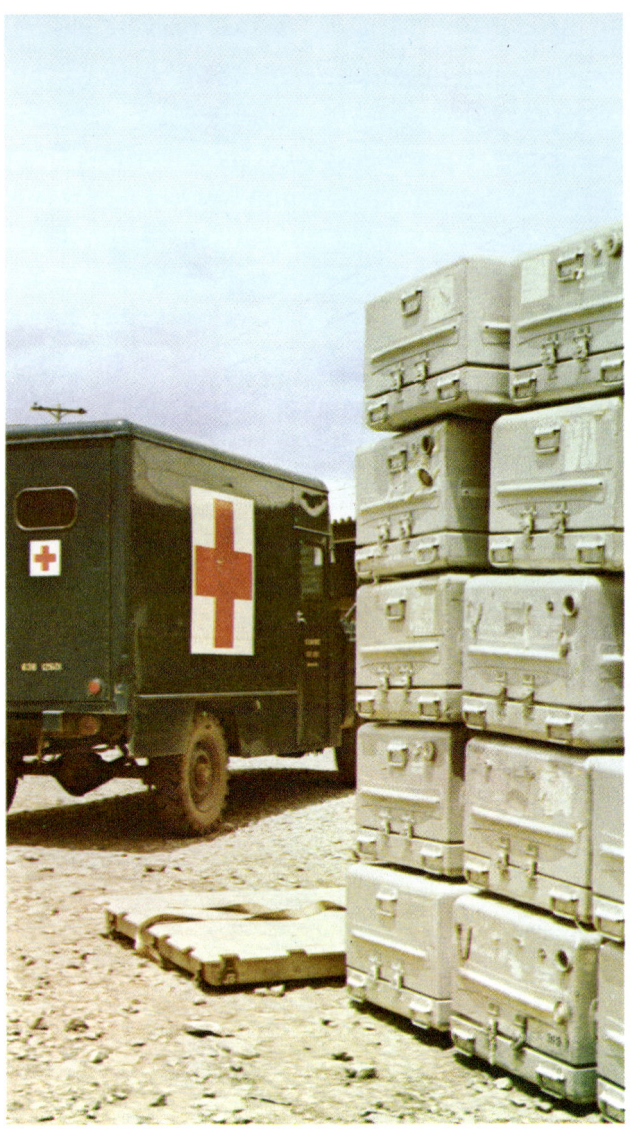

"36 Americans killed in sporadic action..." It was a statistic. Then I witnessed the reality of that statistic. And for the first time...I wept!

remains made the continuation of the procedure unwieldy and it was discontinued.

So remains are shipped out and unloaded as inconspicuously as possible.

Statistics Not Souls

The Colonel in charge of the Mortuary was proud of his job. It is a most difficult one. But all along the line I found people were statistic indoctrinated.

Elaborate charts were shown me showing how in 1961 they handled 3 dead in Vietnam conflict to a record high of 6410 processed in 1966 at Tan San Nuit.

They had the entire operation down to a timed science, alloting so many minutes for each operation from positive identification of remains to final packing. With the high casualty rate such efficiency was demanded. And by reading the newspapers they could pretty well predict their workload for the ensuing few days.

Outside, row upon row, were the aluminum shipping containers stacked high to save space. Outside also were the bloodied and muddied stretchers and bags fresh in from the field. And inside, the overpowering smell of disinfectant and the still and quiet dead. I was given the tour and I was sick—sick of the melo-dramatic painting of the glories of war on TV—sick of the slanted news reports that fail to honestly reveal the horrors of war and the impossibility of the present conflict.

I Wept

As I passed the filled aluminum containers ready to fly back to the States, I read the tags affixed to each one. They were just names—statistics back home—casualties that were described by the top Army echelon as "light."

But they didn't seem "light" to me.

And for the first time—I wept!

They were devastatingly heavy casualties, for this name tag would represent a sorrowful family at home, the loss of a father or a husband forever.

Thirty people in a few days would gather at a grave somewhere in the United States. Few people would be affected. Few would notice.

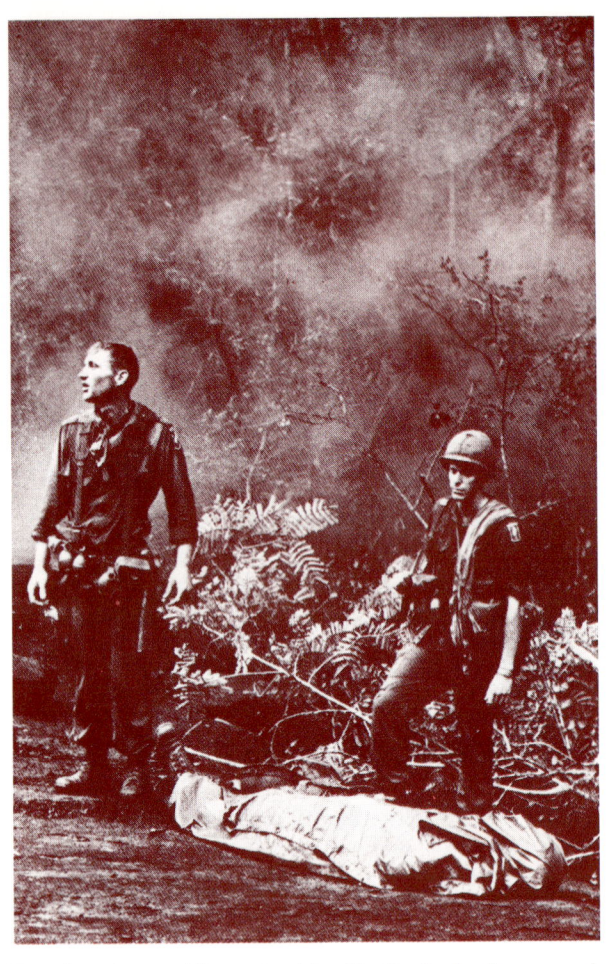

Two American soldiers stand beside the body of a comrade in Vietnam. For him...the war is over.

People would still riot in the streets seeking a handout from Uncle Sam instead of gearing their activities to constructive action.

Flag wavers would still be shouting the glories of war and our cause to fight communism in Vietnam.

Congressmen would still be making inspection tours as part of their travel vacation.

And the leaders of our government would still keep their political ear to the ground, couching their statement in glowing generalities of praise.

But for the dead, there were no blaring trumpets in the hot, steaming, soggy, cow grass where they fell—just the buzz of a multitude of insects—and an end in the blazing sun 10,000 miles from their home. Soon they were whisked to an "off limits" restricted one-story building. (I had to secure permission from two different authorities to go through.)

And finally under the cover of darkness they were flown home.

For them the fight is over.

And the Americans, complaining because an important news event pre-empted their soap opera, or favorite TV comedy, can go back to laughing and enjoying life, taking every opportunity to be a flag waver.

Because for them the Glory is in the living.

And contrary to Memorial Day orators . . . the dead will soon be forgotten.

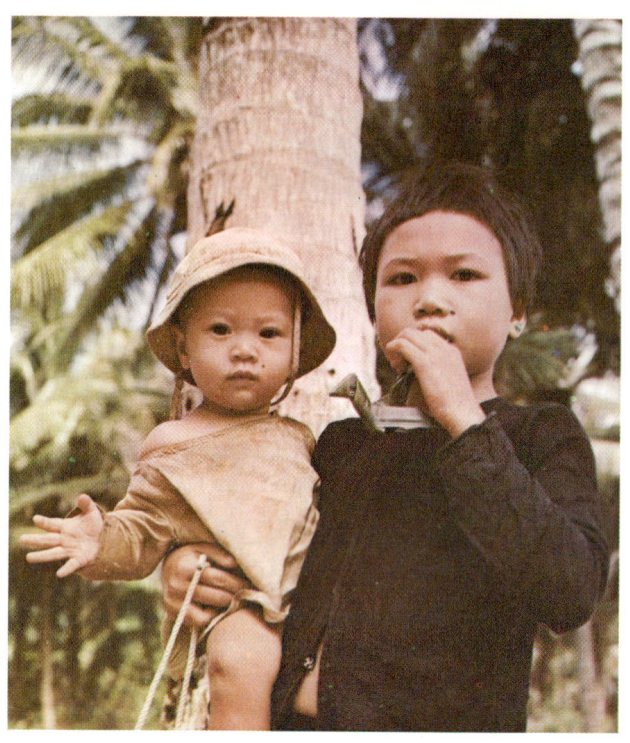

Children are often the innocent victims of war. I came across these two Vietnamese children outside a hospital in Nha Trang. With nothing to their name but the clothes on their back they appeared contented in what they had. At a very early age this girl assumed the responsibility of caring for her little brother. Her biggest joy appears to be the sugarcane bird she made which adds a little sweetness to the bitter realities of life.

CAN MISSIONS FLOURISH IN A LAND AT WAR?

"If we had sent over just one million dollars to support missionary effort in Vietnam . . . this war could have been averted."

This was the statement made by one Air Force Chaplain in Saigon. And other Chaplains and missionaries serving in Vietnam confirmed this belief.

I had viewed the huge U.S. war arsenal of defense here in Vietnam and was quite surprised to learn that in the midst of conflict missionary stations were still operating.

Catholic Churches flourish in this country but a few denominational works exist as well. By far the largest and oldest missionary endeavor in Vietnam is that conducted by The Christian Missionary Alliance Church.

The Alliance compound sits on a hill overlooking the harbor of Nha Trang. Well built, stone-structured buildings are quite spacious and offer the visitor a sharp contrast from the abject poverty at the base of the hill with the fine accommodations in the Alliance compound. It is a welcome relief, and the cool breezes of the sea sweep across this area giving a refreshing uplift as you survey miles of Vietnam from this commanding view.

This mission cooperates with several inter-related works

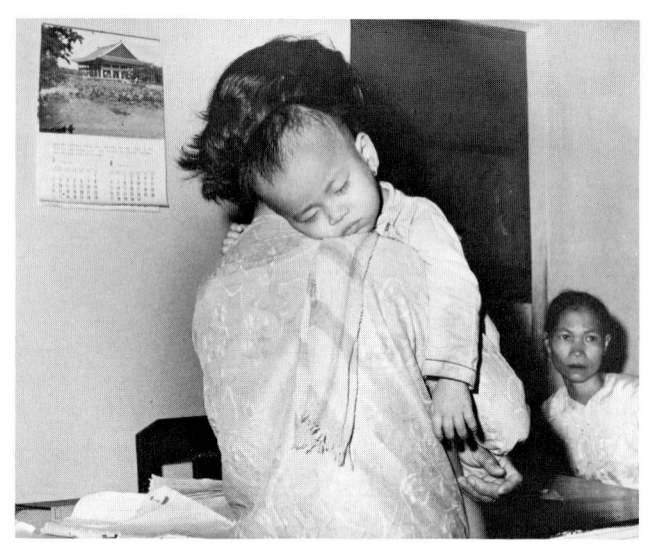

Two Billion Dollars a month fed the machinery of war in Vietnam while little was invested in the "milk of human kindness."

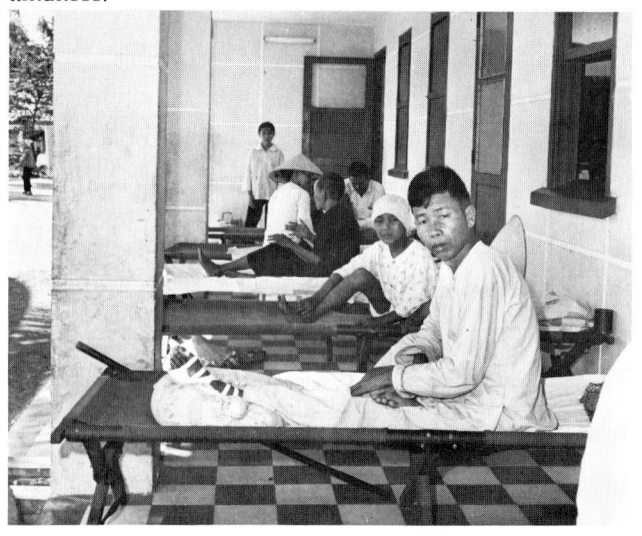

Overcrowded and understaffed hospitals were a way of life in Vietnam and some had to lay outside.

all situated in the same area. Down at the bottom of the hill is the Evangelical Clinic Hospital. It is supported by the Vietnam Christian Service which is a combination of the Mennonite Central Committee, Church World Service and Lutheran World Relief.

The Mennonite Central Committee started this Clinic in cooperation with the Protestant Church in Vietnam in 1960. I found that the word "Protestant" used in Vietnam was equivalent to Evangelical in the States.

It was this Committee that sent doctors and nurses here. Then 1 1/2 years ago, Church World Service and Lutheran World Relief joined in this work . . . plus a hospital in Pleiku and in Saigon.

At that time there were 2 American doctors and 4 American nurses working in this hospital. Their usual term of service is 2 years.

Basically the main work here is in two different areas — tuberculosis and eye surgery. While there, we witnessed an eye operation.

A Haven Of Help

Under U.S. standards the conditions of this Clinic would be considered intolerable. Patients live in the hallway, out on the porch, with their family huddled around them in what appears to be far from antiseptic surroundings. Except in dire circumstances the clinic does not provide any meals for patients. This is the responsibility of their family. Outside I saw an old woman squatting on the ground boiling a concoction of pork and vegetable in an old pot on a little makeshift fire, while nearby someone else was mincing vegetables. Nearby was a bottle of what to the Vietnamese is their steak sauce. It could have knocked you over.

The heat and humidity are oppressive, and in the hospital you see children and women fanning their loved ones to keep them cool and keep off the flies.

In one small room was a mother with a new born babe in a wicker basket. Throughout the hospital were little tots walking around, some only 5 or 6 years of age carrying their brothers or sisters who were only 2 or 3.

The one room that was air-conditioned was the operating room.

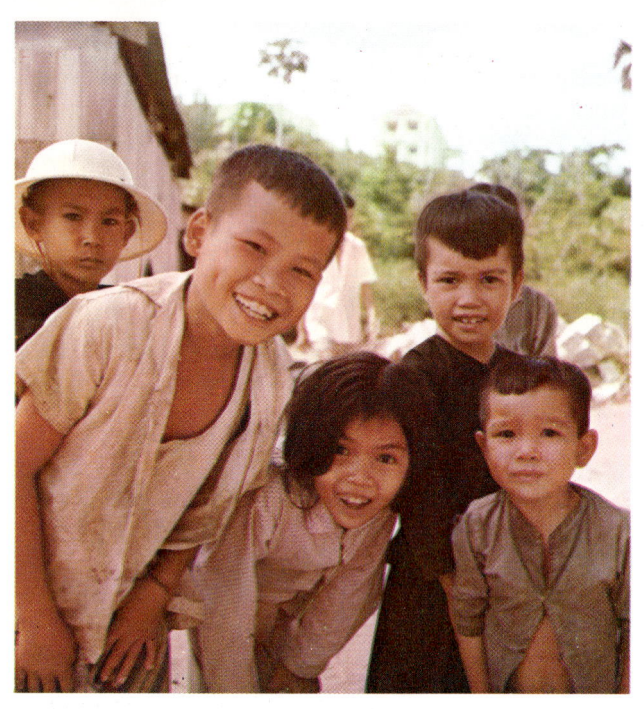

Vietnamese children outside a hospital in Nha Trang, Vietnam.

The work at this clinic is purely social. But every day a missionary from the Alliance comes down to do evangelistic work.

It seems odd that such a hospital and missionary endeavor could exist in the midst of a war zone. But the doctor I interviewed said that as far as he knew he had never had any contact with the VC. It is believed, however, that they probably inadvertently treated VC as there is no real way to differentiate between them.

The clinic handles very few war cases. The clinic is on 2 1/2 acres of land and is actually part of the Protestant Church of Vietnam which consists of an Orphanage (Christian Children's Fund), the clinic and the Alliance school.

The clinic treats about 200 patients a day in their outclinic. They conduct about 6 cataract operations in the week, plus a dozen other cases.

Dr. Linford K. Gehman and Dr. Harold E. Kraybill were the two resident physicians at the clinic. Both are Mennonites from the United States.

While there were 36 beds in the clinic, additional cots, stretchers, and floor mats accommodated many more. Three adjacent structures house an additional 60 tuberculosis patients. Presently 15 Vietnamese interpreters, nurses and nurses aids are employed.

From the clinic I drove up the winding dirt road to the top of the hill where I interviewed Spencer and Barbara Sutherland, missionaries under the Christian & Missionary Alliance Church.

The Alliance work in Vietnam has been in existence over 60 years and there are 4 couples engaged in the work in Nha Trang. Two of the families teach in the Alliance School, which is a Protestant Seminary. Here young Vietnamese men are trained in a 5 year course to be pastors.

They come to the Seminary for two years and then go away from the school for 2 years to open new churches and assist Pastors in remote areas of Vietnam. Then they return to the Seminary for a year and then they are appointed to a Church as a Pastor.

Called To Be Faithful

For 50 years the only missionary group in Vietnam was the Alliance.

These new Pastors were sent out by their own committee with the Alliance acting more as advisors. The decision making is left to the Vietnamese, and in fact the work is an indigenous ministry. Each year 10 to 15 pastors graduate from the Seminary. Because of the war, in the last 5 years only about 50 pastors have gone out in the field.

The war has made it harder for them to succeed because some pastors have to go out and leave their families back in a safe area.

Mrs. Sutherland, remarking on the success of the missionary work, said, "Our work with the Montagard people of Vietnam has been particularly successful. The missionaries who work with them have gone into these villages where the Gospel has been spread and never do they find that the VC have infiltrated . . . but they certainly do come into the villages where the Gospel has not been prevalent. In fact, my husband went on a trip 20 or 30 miles from here and he was advised by military advisors he couldn't stay there at night because it was not a secure area."

"Why is it that the Viet Cong don't bother you, particularly since you are in a war area?"

Mrs. Sutherland replied, "We have not been bothered. They know we're here, I am sure. And if we were going to be of any use to them, perhaps we would be bothered. We have only had one incident in our mission, Ban Me Thuot area, where we had the VC come into our Leprosarium. They kidnapped our woman doctor and male missionary and a young agricultural advisor. That was five years ago and no substantial word has ever been received of their fate."

"Was there ever any missionary work done in North Vietnam?" I asked.

"Yes, we had a quite a bit of work going on right in Hanoi up until the Second World War. Then our missionaries were evacuated. Those who weren't, spent the war in concentration camps."

"Are there Christians now in North Vietnam?"

"Well, definitely, we have word filter down now and then from Christians up there. They don't make any remarks concerning the political situation because they would endanger their lives."

The Absence Of Morality

The general impression many missionaries have of the Vietnamese people is that they think of themselves first. Their existence has not been easy. They have had to struggle for everything they ever got. They don't understand the American altruistic feelings at all (this is true of Vietnamese Christians as well). Americans want to do something good for people, but the Vietnamese don't feel this way. They think the Americans are just a little bit odd . . . a little simple-minded because they always want to give something away.

"I find," I continued, "that in this Hands Across the Sea U.S. handout program that many of the goods and food that come to Vietnam free is either sold back to the U.S. Army at inflated prices or sold back even to their own people who are supposed to get this free. Apparently they have no compunctions as far as morality on their part. Is this true?"

"No compunctions at all," Mrs. Sutherland replied. "They think it is very smart if they can get away with it. No, their conscience would never bother them."

"Do you think the average Vietnamese is concerned about the war or the ideals of fighting communism or making Vietnam free for democracy?" I asked.

"Some are, but others are more concerned about whether they are going to have to serve in the Army. We have had 2 or 3 students taken right off a bus and put into the Army. I don't think they have a patriotism as we know it. The major religions are Catholicism and Buddhism. Protestants represent a very small percent. They have no central point of loyalty because they don't trust anybody else. This seems to be indicative of the Vietnamese culture, and it will take several generations to change this."

Body Counts

"We read about the body counts of so many hundreds of VC killed and usually by the end of the week, the body count of VC comes to the thousands," I remarked.

"Well, when they say VC . . . after you've been here a while

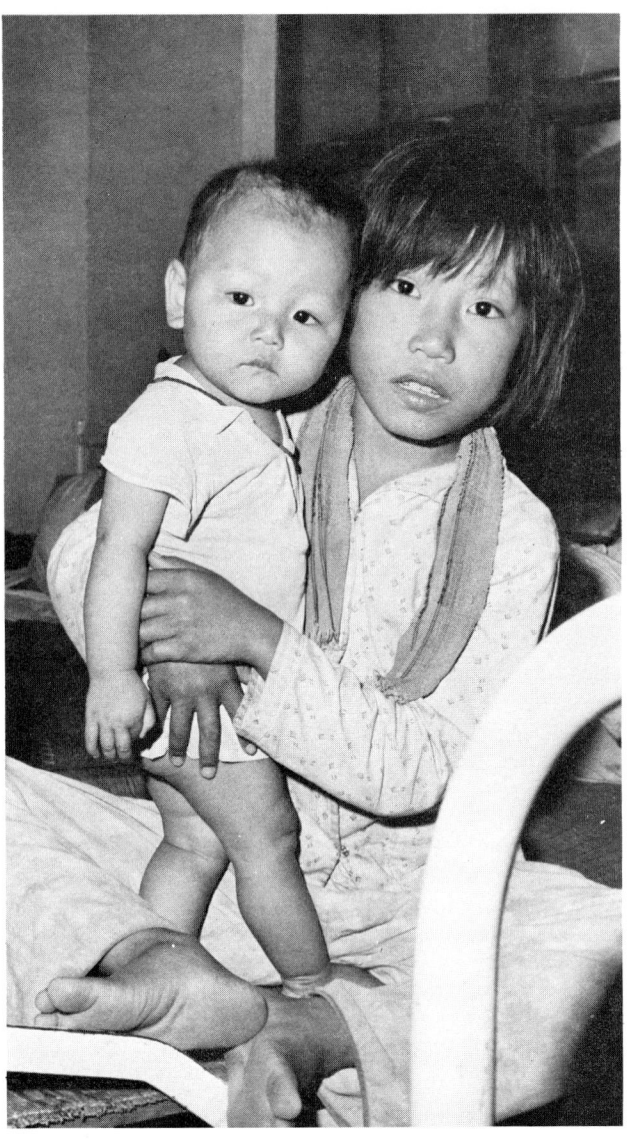

War is the only way of living they know . . . and you can see it in the faces of the Vietnamese children, especially in the hospitals.

you must realize that they could not all be VC. Maybe they were in the wrong area at the time. Many innocent people have been killed just because they are Vietnamese. Why, we can't tell VC from non-VC and we've lived here nine years," Mrs. Sutherland replied.

Mrs. Sutherland told of seeing bombings going on just a few miles from their mission station the day before I interviewed her. However, it is the policy of the mission not to know what's going on and remain as much as possible nonpolitical.

"What do you see for Viet Nam five or ten years from now?" I asked.

"I don't know, but I do know the United States can't impose upon the Vietnamese the type of government we have. The Vietnamese don't think like we do in too many ways. They don't trust each other. I don't know even if they could ever have free election. I would assume that the same thing would happen here as took place in Korea—a continuing police action."

Mrs. Sutherland concluded her remarks by saying that more missionaries were needed in Vietnam to carry on the work.

Many Americans were unaware that the United States was spending over two billion dollars a month to fight a war in Vietnam that cost over 50,000 American lives.

No one knows what would have happened if just one million dollars had been expended for missionary activities instead. One thing is certain, military might alone has not resolved the Vietnam problem.

THE CHAPLAIN . . . SPIRITUAL COUNSELOR AND MOTHER

The Chaplain's life is a busy one.

Lt. Col. Walter Huber of the United States Air Force was responsible for a religious program for 13,000 Air Force personnel in Tan San Nuit Air Base in Saigon.

The emphasis of the Chaplain's duties has shifted somewhat from the era of World War II days.

The familiar scene of a Chaplain talking to a group of pilots just before they go to strike their mission is no longer evident.

Here, pilots fly around the clock, sometimes only one or two at a time. Because of this, a dual emphasis is placed on the Flight Line Ministry and Single Airman Ministry.

In the Flight Line Ministry Chaplains go where their men are and offer spiritual counsel. And in the Single Airman Ministry much of their time is devoted to counselling with individual airmen.

Lt. Col. Huber, from Houston, Texas, is a graduate of Concordia Seminary with 16 years of service in the Air Force. He supervised five services a week conducted under his command.

Chaplains in every branch of the service have a wide degree of latitude in what they can preach. Most Protestant

Chaplains do not get involved in specific doctrines of their Church but outside of this, no restrictions are placed on them. They are allowed to preach just as they would in their own Church back home.

Chaplains from each denomination are determined by a general rule of thumb of one Chaplain for every 100,000 membership in that denomination.

Sometimes they are required to be on call 24 hours a day.

War And Marriage

At 1 AM the day before I arrived, an airman called the Chaplain. His voice was choking with tears. He had just received a letter from home with divorce papers in it.

Chaplains find that the strain of family separation, homesickness and pending divorce action are the main problems confronting our servicemen when they seek a Chaplain. And contrary to popular belief, usually it is the woman back home who proves the unfaithful one.

In World War II this trend worked in reverse, however.

The Armed Services had very strict guidelines on when a soldier could be returned home from Vietnam because of compassionate reasons. Pending divorce problems are not sufficient reason for a soldier to get a 30 day pass to return to the United States . . . that is unless the Chaplain feels that by returning, the marriage can be resolved. Oftentimes, however, after the soldier went home and they kissed and made up, as soon as he returned to Vietnam, the wife again became unfaithful.

The environment that soldiers lived in Vietnam was not conducive to resolving problems either.

Saigon, where many servicemen were stationed, was once a beautiful city. But from 1957 one million people have migrated down to Saigon from the North and the city has quickly deteriorated to streets of filth and overcrowded conditions.

Right and wrong don't mean much to Vietnamese people. Many were stealing U.S. servicemen blind and they had no respect for human life. The Chaplains I interviewed felt that the Vietnamese were not a nation of people, but rather splinter groups with no sense of loyalty.

And it is within this environment that the U.S. soldier

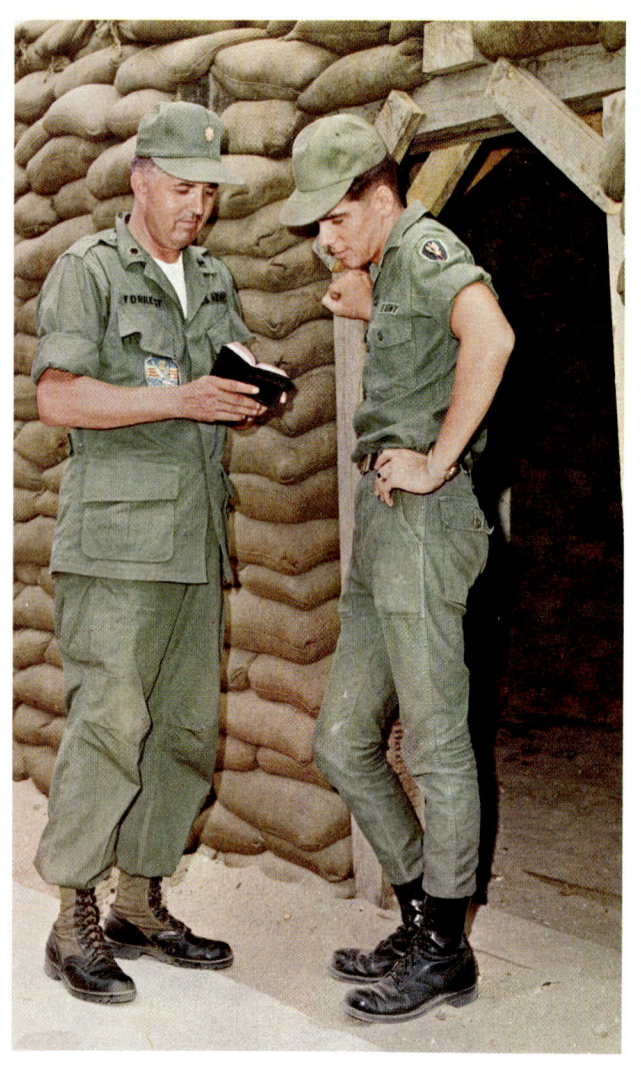

Dennis with dedicated Chaplain Forrest.

found himself . . . an environment that created many problems that the Chaplain must resolve.

The situation was not helped either by the indifference shown back home even in evangelical churches.

The Forgotten War

One chaplain related that he had been in Vietnam 5 months and his wife reported that not once in these five months had her Pastor had prayer for the servicemen from their Church serving in Vietnam.

Nor was there any prayer for peace. She suggested to her Pastor that the following Sunday they have prayer. He obliged and then remarked, "That's a good idea; we ought to do it again sometime."

This lack of interest disturbed most Chaplains in Vietnam, particularly when they faced every day the cold realities of war.

Also discouraging in many instances was the lack of mail our servicemen received. It's hard for people to imagine how much servicemen look forward to receiving mail from home.

I didn't appreciate this myself until I spent 10 days in Viet Nam and each day anxiously awaited Mail Call . . . which is usually twice a day. And when a letter didn't come, a feeling of loneliness crept in. The dull day-to-day routine in an oppressively hot and humid country, living under primitive conditions, can best be alleviated by parents and loved ones back home sending letters and packages at regular intervals. If this were done, Chaplains feel their job would have been much easier.

From Saigon I went to Nha Trang where I interviewed another chaplain.

He had just arrived in Vietnam from a successful Chaplain's work at the Army Processing Center in Fort Lewis, Washington.

On the evening of a service in Fort Lewis, the Chaplain would go through the barracks inviting soldiers to attend. After the service they would have coffee and doughnuts. On his first Sunday he had 6 people. But by the time he left for Vietnam this group had grown to over 130 people. No soldier is kept in Fort Lewis for more than 48 hours—

since all of them are enroute to overseas posts . . . mostly Vietnam.

"While I wouldn't preach baptism by immersion, I would get into the fact that I believe in the eternal security of the believer," the Chaplain remarked. "In fact, in personal work you are only limited as you would limit yourself."

"This, I find is a real fruitful field because here they are thinking in terms of eternity because people are being killed around them all the time."

Chaplains generally do not get out into battle areas. They do go to the field aid stations when the men are being brought back. And this is really the ideal place for the Chaplain to be.

God, Sex And Patriotism

"I notice the Armed Services have an entertainment program which is really diametrically opposed to what the Chaplain is attempting to accomplish," I remarked. "I took some pictures and tape recorded a couple of these shows. Some of the performers mixed God, Sex and Patriotism all in the same breath, the beer and liquor flowed freely. This type of performance, including burlesque, seems to pervade more . . . almost nightly . . . than the services the Chaplain provides."

"Well, this is true from the standpoint that many of the shows that come over are based on the sex angle," the Chaplain replied. "But the Chaplain has to do his job from the standpoint that he must preach the Gospel and bring man to God. He can't sit back and say, Well, there's going to be a U.S.O. show and what good will my preaching do! The Lord has promised to bless His word and our job is to preach. This is all we can do. I can't control who comes over."

The Chaplain found that servicemen here were concerned about the total disrespect for the law back home. While here, the Detroit riots were in full swing. One morning at the breakfast table several officers remarked "maybe we should go back home and take care of the United States before we take care of Vietnam."

In Vietnam one of the most distressing facts Chaplains had to cope with was the heavy traffic of prostitutes. In

Nha Trang, as an example, the Chaplain said it is impossible for a GI to walk down the streets of the city without at least being approached 5 to 10 times.

This was a most difficult mission field and never before have so many avenues of sin been so concentrated in a confusing war effort, where the people of the land we came to save in many cases could care less.

This is Vietnam. And for the Chaplain, he found himself face to face on Satan's greatest battle ground. It is a challenge that defies description. And to this Chaplain, Christ was the only answer.

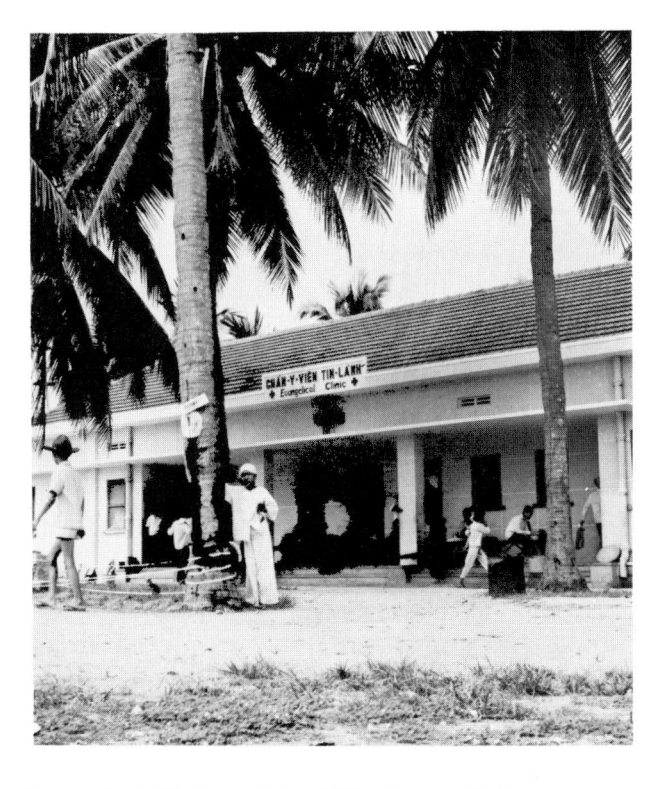

Evangelical Clinic outside of Nha Trang, Vietnam.

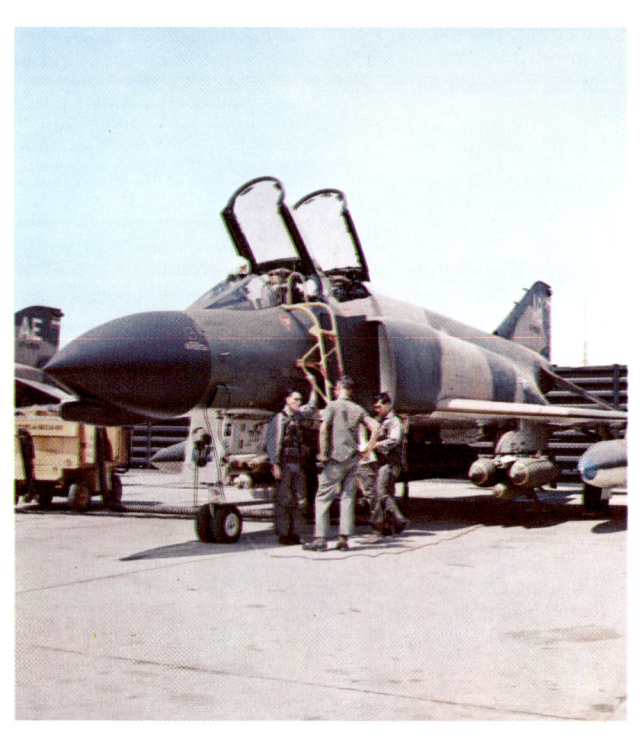

Battle weary pilots prepare for another bombing strike on North Vietnam. Over 3700 airplanes and over 4800 helicopters were lost in the Vietnam war!

FAINT AT ATTENTION

The next seven days with my son were thrilling ones. One could never escape the heat and the dust and the ever present war but these seemed minor for father and son were together.

In the barracks huge floor fans were reversed and hung from the wooden ceiling and they ran all day and all night. It was a welcome relief even though the air they fanned was hot.

The bases operated on one of three conditions: White (all clear), YELLOW (stand-by for possible action) and RED (be prepared to defend).

One night in the barracks we had just come back from the enlisted men's club with a soft drink and a hot dog. It was midnight. Half the men were asleep, others were watching the Armed Forces TV.

Yellow Alert

Suddenly a sergeant came running in the barracks announcing YELLOW ALERT. I had no idea what was going on and was pretty tired from the activities of that day. Many G.I.'s had just come off their guard duty stints and were looking forward to getting some sleep. It was a real comedy to watch. Groans and gripes prevailed through the barracks as exhausted G.I.'s got out of their bunks and started dressing. On Yellow alert they had to get dressed in their full combat gear including tin bucket (the 4 1/2 pound camouflaged helmet), rifle and rifle clip belt, canteen and jungle boots.

Twenty minutes later we were still shaking one G.I. trying to get him out of bed. After getting in full gear no one seemed to know what to do. Most of them just flopped down on their bed. One thing was for sure, I didn't know what to do. Finally someone turned the lights out. Somebody thought it would be a good idea. We were real sitting targets. After about a half hour they thought it might be a good idea to line up in formation outside. Another half hour and they were back turning in their rifles.

We still didn't know what happened and I guess I looked rather silly—a lonely civilian sitting on a cot alone in the barracks wondering whether I should head for the nearest sandbagged bunker or wave a flag out the window like Barbara Fritchie.

They told me the first night they had a Yellow Alert the G.I.'s spent half the night groping in the dark looking for their assigned bunker.

A Colonel at Da Nang, where my son and I visited a few days later, told me when Viet Cong mortar fire destroyed about 65 million dollars worth of planes there a few weeks earlier . . . over half the casualties were G.I.'s falling out of bed bumping arms, legs and heads.

When in Saigon they told me I would need a PX pass to enter the PX at any base. I didn't have time to wait the required 4 days for this pass to be processed. My son wanted to take me to the local PX on base in Nha Trang. What to do about a pass? Fortunately there was a Vietnamese guard at the PX door. So each day I passed through I would wave a card—a credit card, social security card, anything that looked official. It worked—much to my son's amazement.

It wasn't that we didn't appreciate the food slugged on the World War II steel trays at the G.I. mess hall but we wanted something more appetizing.

Getting A Good Hamburger

Practically every evening about 5 PM we would hitchhike to the Air Force Base about 4 miles down the road. Hitch hiking a ride is the standard mode of transportation in Vietnam and most everyone picks you up. Many a time my son and I rode in jeeps, open trucks, paneled trucks with privates, captains, sergeants and colonels. Jumping up on tailgates got to be quite an art and we joked constantly about the poor limousine service we were receiving in Vietnam.

The Air Force cafeteria had food that was closest to that of home and the prices were reasonable. One could get a steak, a real honest-to-goodness hamburger, a milk shake or hot dog. And the orange and grape drinks loaded with crushed ice in extra large drinking cups were out of this world. With so much heat and humidity one perspires almost constantly and it is unbelievable what large quantities of liquids can be consumed at one sitting. Nothing was quite as refreshing as the ice filled orange drinks.

Meeting A General

One evening my son's chaplain invited us to meet with a group of officers of the First Field Headquarters who were to have an informal session with General William K. Harrison. General Harrison was the Chief U.N. Delegate to the Panmunjon Peace Conference in Korea in 1953.

Dennis I am sure was awed by the occasion. Here he was a lonely Private First Class surrounded by the top brass of First Corps—Captains, Majors, Colonels and a General. I guess they too wondered what he was doing there. So I brought my camera equipment—put some in his hands so he would look important. He still felt rather hesitant so I said, "After all they're only human. And don't forget they are working for me because it's my taxes that's paying their salary."

That seemed to put his mind at ease and the session began. General Harrison began by telling a little of his own experiences in the Army, how he had grown up in the ranks to the status of a General.

He related some of the problems he was faced with and how he handled them.

He then opened the discussion for questions from the floor. None of us was prepared for the question that followed.

To Kill Or Not To Kill

A colonel stood up and said, "As a military leader we are called on at one time or another to directly kill or indirectly kill somebody by shooting or by commanding someone else

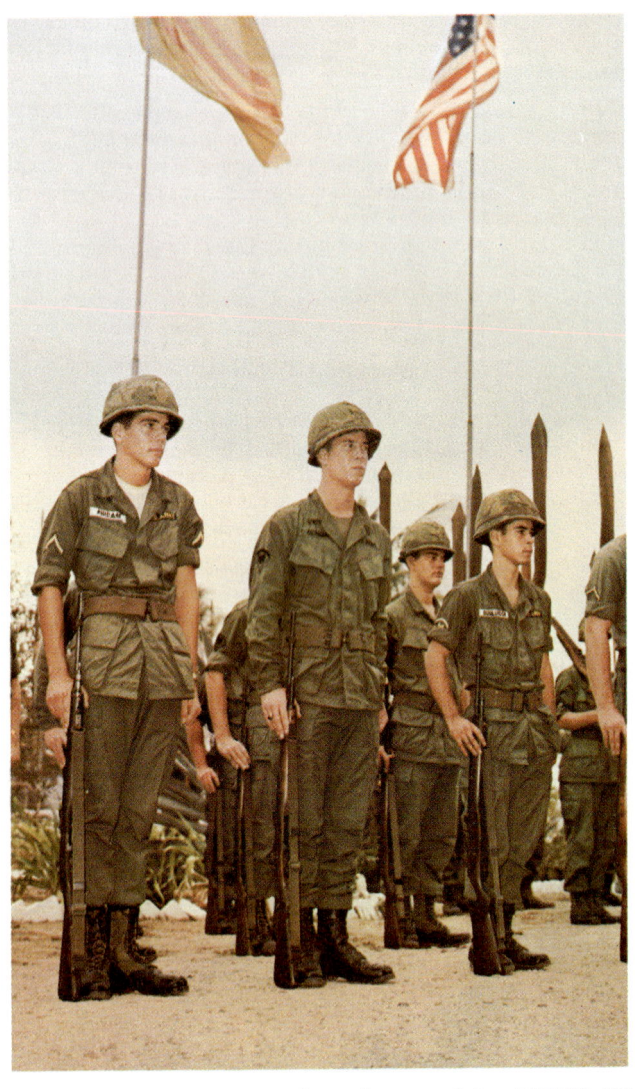

"...and for heaven's sake, if you have to faint, FAINT AT ATTENTION!" (Dennis is at left in photograph at change of command ceremony.)

to shoot. I must confess this has been a constant problem with me. How do you as a General with a firm belief in the tenents of the Bible reconcile this?"

"Well," General Harrison replied, "I had to face this issue long ago. In the late Twenties I used to get pamphlets put out by the Methodist Church and the Episcopal Church which, if they were right, I was no better than a murderer—so I said, 'Well, Harrison, you better find out because if this is right, you better get out of the service.'"

"So I figured if there is an answer it must be in the Bible. I believe the Bible is the Word of God. I read the verse which says, 'thou shalt not kill' and some believe you can't even kill a fly. This however refers to murder. I also realized the Bible says 'love your enemy.' I agree. But I had to appreciate the fact that in war a crime has already been made—an act of aggression. One can't avoid the choice. It is impossible to evade this. Either you're going to protect your country or you're just going to say 'I don't believe in killing' and then say 'go ahead, buddy, help yourself.'

"I remember several years ago reading a magazine where a leading clergyman said the Church must find a third position—in the middle. But the point is there is no third position. It's just this—you're alive—you're a citizen of some country. When your country is at war, the capability of your country to wage this war is the sum of all the coordinated effort of the citizens. You may not have very much to offer but what you have is real. And to the extent that you deprive your country of it—you are giving it to the enemy. You cannot avoid helping one or the other. There is just no way you can evade this."

I could see my son's eyes light up as the General and top brass discussed real issues of war—issues brought out of discussion that generally would only come out in closed confidential heart to heart meetings.

At the end of the meeting Dennis and I shook hands with the top brass and with General Harrison. As we left we heard him remark to a small group of officers concerning the state of America. "America", he said, "is becoming more of a pagan country and we can't solve a single social problem."

It was an evening well spent and we celebrated it on our cot with a soft drink and cookies which had just arrived from home.

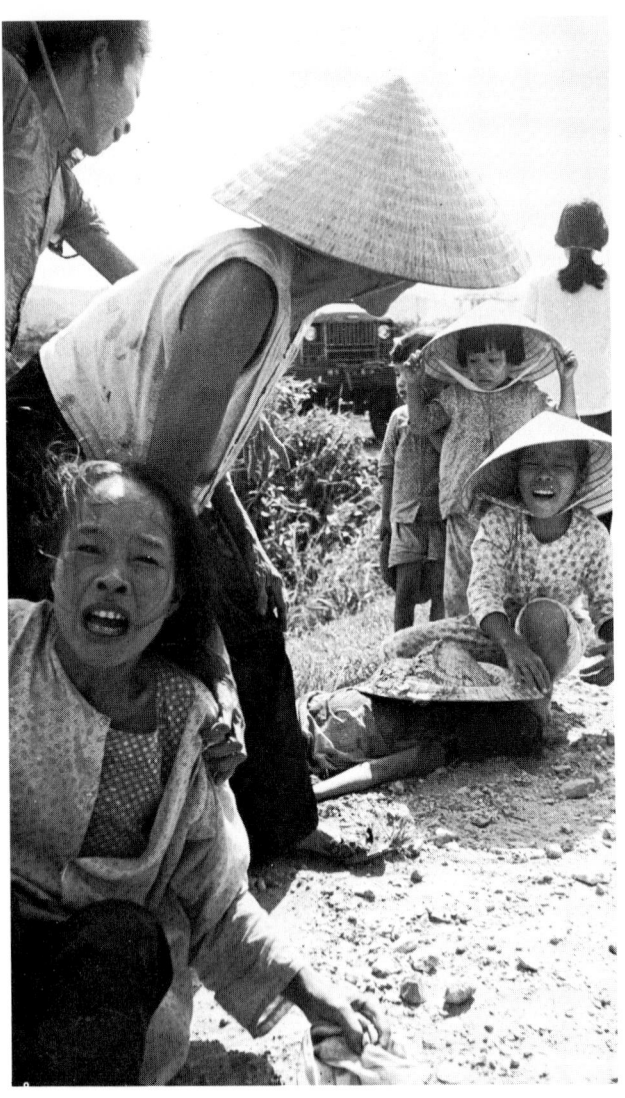

Tragedy is etched on the faces of these Vietnamese women as a mother mercifully places a hat over the body of her dead daughter. The anguish portrayed in this photograph lends credence to the African proverb: "When the elephants go to war, it's the grass that gets trampled!"

Mutt And Jeff

The next day brought rain and an introduction to the monsoon season soon to begin. A change of command ceremony was to take place the following day in front of the administration building of I Field Force Headquarters. Dennis and his sidekick Goggoluchi, the Mutt and Jeff of the Headquarters Company of the 17th Combat Aviation Group, were among the "chosen few" to be in the honor guard.

Dressed in full gear with the steel pot helmet and rifle they boarded the barred windowed bus along with about 40 other G.I.'s and myself. The windows are barred because the Viet Cong had a bad habit of tossing grenades at them causing many casualties. It was drizzling and we were supposed to have about a three hour practice session prepratory for the big day. For an hour we sat in the bus . . . and it rained.

Finally the order was given to proceed and the bus traveled the four miles to I Field Force Headquarters in the rain. And then we sat there another hour as it continued to rain. Good humored griping prevailed as finally the bus returned to our barracks still in the rain. No practice that day.

Early the next morning the bus made the journey again. This time it was cloudy, for which the G.I.'s were thankful For at the actual change of command ceremony that afternoon they would have to stand at attention for about one hour in practice and another hour in the broiling sun as the various brass gave them change of command talks and reviewed the troops. And after a few minutes the heavy steel combat helmet feels like a ton while the perspiration runs in rivulets under your full dress combat uniform. It is not unusual even for hard-nosed sergeants to collapse under the strain.

The captain was barking orders telling the G.I.'s what to expect at the change of command ceremony. This was to be a big one. Even General Westmoreland would be there.

"So remember," he shouted, "Keep that steel pot on your head in one place. Don't wiggle it around. It will only seem heavier. And for heaven's sake, if you have to faint, FAINT AT ATTENTION!"

SAD GOODBYES

The end of my 10 day stay in Vietnam was fast approaching. It had been a wonderful reunion with my son Dennis, serving in the U.S. Army.

I'll never forget, as I am sure he will not, the day I arrived in Nha Trang aboard a C-130 . . . and the happy reunion. He had met me with a jeep and together we rode into town for a steak dinner. As an accredited correspondent, I was entitled officer's quarters and a pass to eat in the officer's dining room. However, to be with my son and also experience the average G.I. living conditions, I chose to live in the barracks and eat in the regular mess hall.

Rank Makes A Difference

Throughout my tour of Vietnam I witnessed a different kind of segregation—the segregation between officer and enlisted man. And while I could appreciate this as an inbred Army tradition, I was dismayed that in many areas, living conditions for enlisted men were more primitive.

I realized that this was war and I didn't mind roughing it. What did bother me was the rank carried unwarranted privileges. They, too, should shoulder the same war, or else the ordinary G.I. should be accorded equal privileges. The brunt of the casualty rate was born by the lowly EM (Enlisted Man) and he also got the short end of the stick.

While officers ate off white table cloths from dishes, the enlisted man stood in line at the mess hall (dining room), picked up a World War II-style tray, and was slung food that in many cases was both unappetizing and short in quantity.

My recollections are still too vivid on the enlisted men's latrines (bathrooms). If any mother back home could have seen them, Congress would have been flooded with mail. I found some filthy with inoperative toilets, many basins with no mirrors, and showers that did not work—or when they did, spilled water and sand all over the floor leaving it in a state of constant quagmire.

In talking to some officers—the segregation is so complete that few officers realize these conditions exist since they have no occasion to share the enlisted man's fare—I know the remark will be made that this is war. But improvements could be made with little cost and just a little more Commanding Officer concern.

An officer is supposed to be a leader, setting a good example. Yet several Chaplains commented to me that few officers attended Chapel each Sunday, and that the Commanding Officer and his Assistant at one base at which I was present never attended. I found some officers more concerned about whether a weary, perspiring enlisted man saluted him as he passed or whether his air conditioner was operating properly.

The Chaplains complained to me that they usually had only one crack at the G.I. each week, Sunday—to get him spiritually straight—while the Army, through the U.S.O., barraged the G.I. almost nightly with questionable shows geared to lower his moral standards. Every show I witnessed was either filled with obscene jokes, half-naked girls, or just plain burlesque.

I witnessed many a G.I. being served unlimited quantities of beer only to be escorted dead-drunk back to his barracks by his buddies.

At the end of my trip to Vietnam, my son and I flew up to Da Nang. Here we witnessed the devasting destruction of the Air Base where a surprise attack by the Viet Cong left $65 million dollars worth of damage. In Westmoreland's oft-phrased "Secure areas" just 6 miles from the base on a grassy plain, the V.C. had launched a mortar barrage 5 minutes long that left millions of dollars in destruction and cost more American lives.

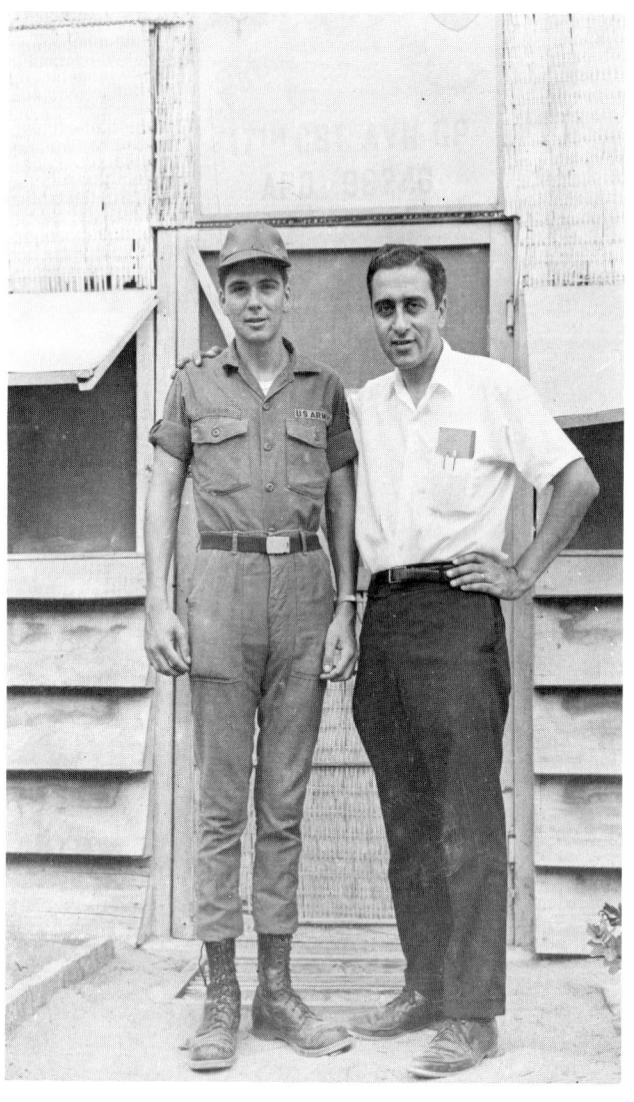

Dennis with father outside his headquarters in Nha Trang, Vietnam.

Returning to Saigon, I boarded an Air America plane, a line chartered by the U.S.

Don't Forget To Write

It was a sad farewell as I said goodbye to my son. And the last word he said as the plane door closed was, "Don't forget to write!"

And for once I know how really important mail is to the G.I. In many areas Mail Call is twice a day every day. And I had found myself anxiously awaiting each Mail Call and going away a little sad when there was no letter for me.

There are many heartaches here—like the G.I. I met whose girl had just written him telling him she married his best friend. That G.I. was drunk for two days.

Youngsters who never smoked or drank find themselves doing so for the first time . . . and under the constant barrage of foul mouth sergeants soon find their language contaminated with the same filth. Many of the service jobs are performed by Vietnamese, which only adds to the utter frustration of living in Vietnam.

Many times I wished that every American could witness what I did in Vietnam, but then I wondered whether it would do any good.

Arriving once more in Saigon, a young Army Colonel picked me up to give me a ride into town.

As many others before, he asked me what I thought about the war. Previously I had refused to comment, but this time I gave him my honest opinion with both barrels.

He wasn't too talkative the rest of the trip.

My personal opinion is that the war in Vietnam was America's costliest mistake which bled Americans at the rate of two billion dollars or more a month and more important over 50,000 American lives.

The State Department went through lengthy explanations to rationalize our commitment to Vietnam, and yet was equally adroit in ignoring commitments in other areas when it was not politically feasible.

In sharp contrast to the filth of Vietnam, I witnessed the cleanliness and unity of the neighboring country of

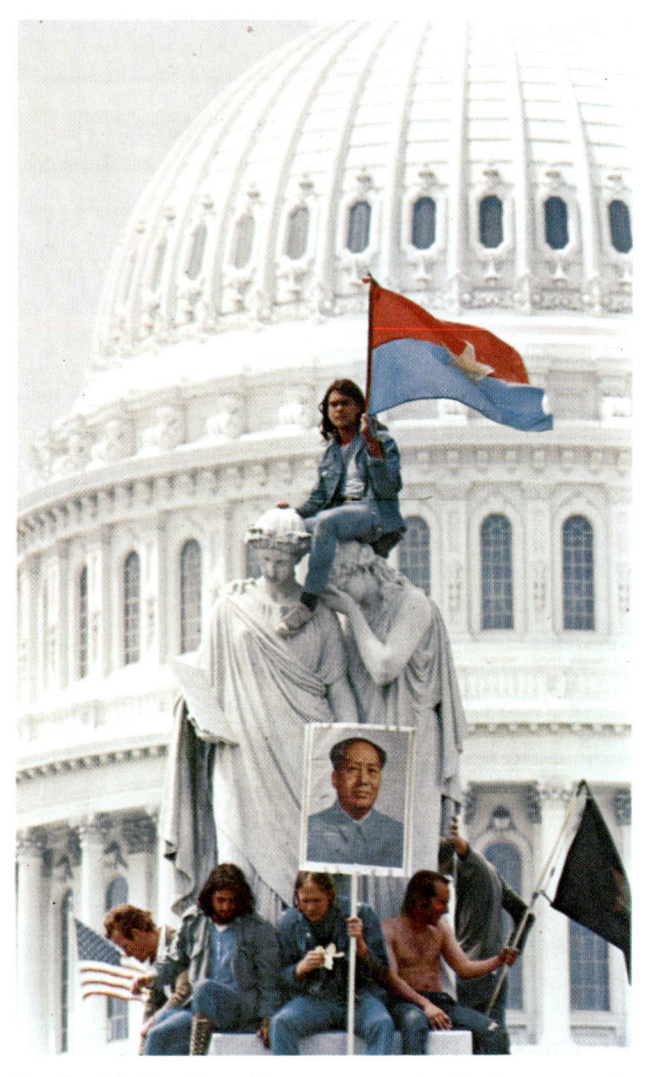

Youth with Viet Cong flag atop statue in Washington, D.C. during height of Vietnam War protests.

Thailand. Here were people with a purpose, living side by side—though with divergent political persuasions.

A Mind To Work

In the Old Testament Nehemiah said the wall of Jerusalem was completed because "the people had a mind to work."

I did not find this true of the people of Vietnam.

Our Government and much of our press said we are fighting so that Vietnam could have a free election, and they point with pride to the current free elections.

If the people in America only realized that nothing could be further from the truth.

If so called "free" Vietnam elections had been held in the United States, this is how they would have been conducted. President Johnson would have gone to Congress and outlawed Goldwater, Nixon and Reagan from running against him because their "views are divergent to the country's interest." Their names would then be removed from the ballot and Johnson would run against lesser candidates who stood no chance of winning.

So Vietnam's five million eligible voters faced a stacked ticket—stacked in favor of the military clique of Ky and Thieu.

In the 1967 Provisional Assembly—under the watchful eye of Ky's National Police Chief—seven of Ky's principal opponents were forbidden to run.

This is the type of Democracy we spawned in Vietnam, laden with graft and corruption.

Here is a country where the poor are really poor, and the rich comfortably rich, and in between lies the filth and degradation that civilization (beginning with the French) has spawned.

It is a country with no central loyalty, with a people who could care less, run by a dictatorial demi-god who has hoodwinked the Americans into paying Vietnam rent for use of its land while we fight its war.

A Hollow Victory

Even though the U.S. achieved a semblance of peace, it was a hollow victory. The phrase "containing Communism" has been used as an excuse of building a complex of military might in Vietnam. This aim is a fine one, but the methods used must be subjected to some serious questioning. Perhaps far fetched as it is—all this effort should have been expended towards a four-lane super highway between Saigon and Hanoi to enable Prime Minister Ky to return to his homeland and provide a free interchange of peoples.

And along the road, American units could have been posted as watch dogs interspersed with Howard Johnson restaurants and good old-fashioned billboards shouting the phrase I found on the walls of the Hospital Casualty ward, "TELL GOD YOU LOVE HIM."

Far fetched? Perhaps. But not any more far fetched than our present methods.

I witnessed a little America here in Viet Nam—huge complexes of buildings and concrete runways everywhere I went—all geared for the massive destruction of war. And it seemed like a lion fighting a mouse, and somehow the mouse, small and insignificant as it was, created a reign of terror and death.

Statistics Not Love

The Army flooded me with statistics on their air and ground force might—even down to the minute on how long it takes to embalm a fallen G.I. and get him home.

We geared ourselves to the arsenal of war. How much more rewarding—though admittedly more difficult—if we had used the same ingenuity and techniques to gear ourselves to the arsenal of peace.

Many confided to me that, sad as it is to admit, America is geared to an economy of war, and the leeches of greed use all their talents to extract top dollar from the grief of war.

And while I sat writing this in Bangkok, the Bangkok Post daily printed on its front page a running account of "U.S. Riots at a Glance." A $40 million rat control bill is laughingly voted down by the House while the President says, "I have no doubt whatever, our country will be able to do whatever is necessary to meet the problems of cost to eliminate the cause of rats."

While we were minding other people's business 10,000 miles away, we are falling apart at the seams back home.

I was present at a meeting held for a handful of Army officers at the I Corps Headquarters in Nha Trang, Viet Nam.

The speaker was Retired General W. K. Harrison (U.S. representative at the Korean Truce).

His concluding remarks were: "America is becoming more and more a pagan country and we have not solved and cannot solve a single social problem."

Is it not a wonder that our G.I.'s in Vietnam—almost to the man—had their own calendar where they daily crossed off the days, looking forward to the end of their year's duty when at least they can "Get back to the world."

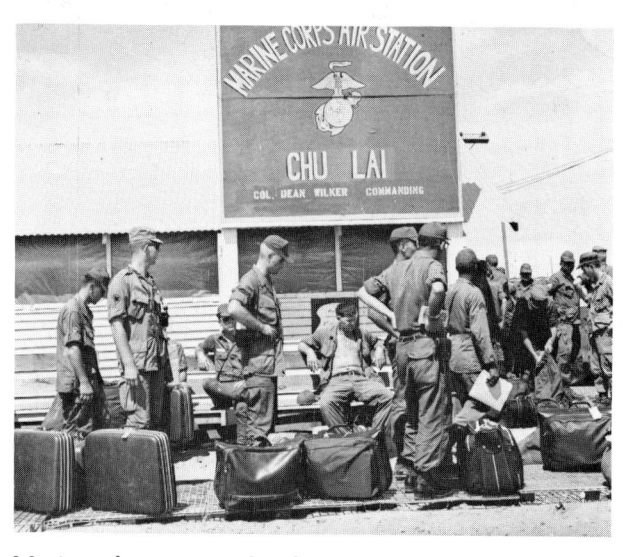

Marines, having completed one year of duty in Vietnam, anxiously line up at Chu Lai air base in Vietnam in preparation for the long flight home.

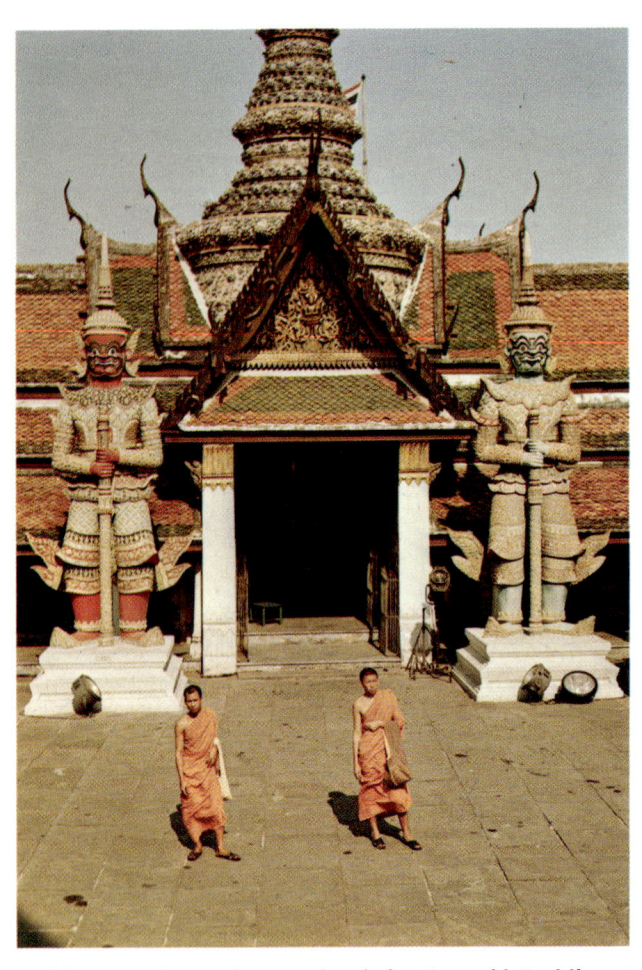

Buddhist monks at the temple of the Emerald Buddha at Bangkok, Thailand. This is one of the great shrines in Southeast Asia. Buddhists believe in many demons and spirits, like this guardian spirit in the same temple.

IS THERE NO BALM IN GILEAD?

From the dead American in Viet Nam to the dying in Calcutta I was about to witness the living dead in Jordan.

From Viet Nam I flew to Bangkok where I spent a day sightseeing and relaxing after a hectic 10 day stay in a country at war. It was a most welcome relief and a sharp contrast from the filth and run-down conditions of Vietnam. Here in Bangkok there were super highways; the streets were clean and living standards high.

The Thais have a King but are run on a constitutional government. They have a deep sense of loyalty to their country and effectively quell any attempts at communist infiltration from the North. Unlike Vietnam, they have a high moral code. The Prime Minister has banned Playboy Magazine from the country and banned mini-skirts from appearing on television. He even went so far as forbidding students and government officials from wearing mini-skirts to schools and offices.

Luh Muang, the Prime Minister, commented that it is the responsibility of the adults to guide the younger generation towards a clean and healthy life. What a refreshing and welcome change this was compared to the attitude of most Americans!

Leaving Thailand I flew through the night, arriving in Beirut at dawn.

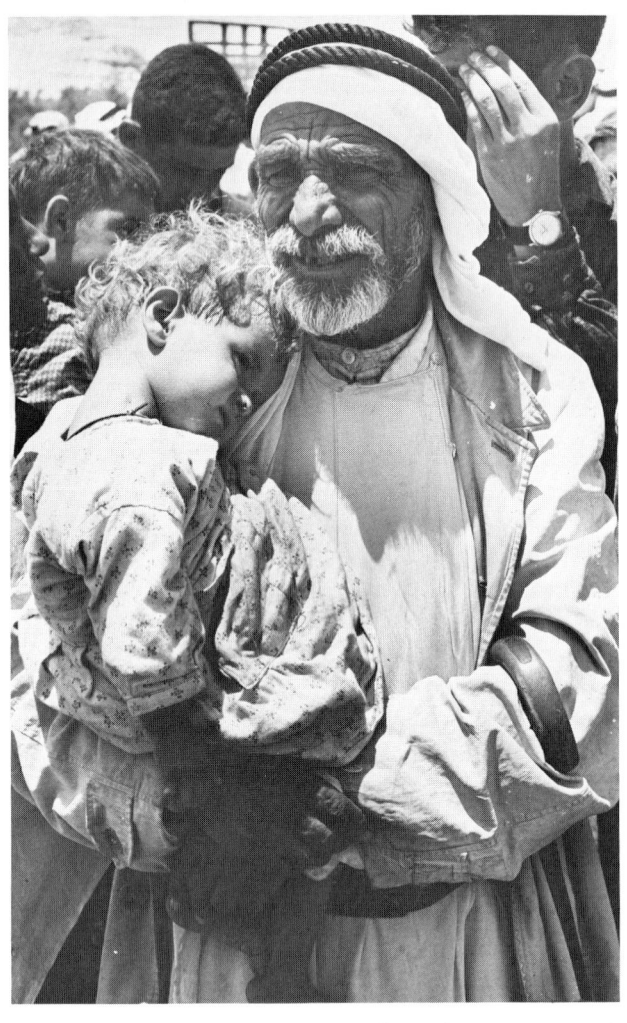

Unaware of the tragedy around him this young Arab refugee sleeps peacefully in the weary arms of his grandfather.

Beautiful Beirut

Both my parents were from Lebanon, and it was a thrill to come, for the first time, to the homeland of my mother and father. I found the climate and landscape of Beirut beautiful, nestled at the mouth of blue Mediterranean Sea.

Because my time was limited, I wanted to see some of the historic spots, and my driver-guide drove me 50 miles to Baalbak, often termed an "ancient paradise."

Here in the middle of the desert are the remains of what once was a proud city; now just a few high pillars mark the horizon. Legend has it that Adam lived in Baalbak.

As you stand in these ruins and see the carvings and inscriptions well preserved in this arid sunny climate, it is difficult to believe that these structures and artifacts were built about 12 A.D. or possibly during the reign of Julius Caesar.

From there my driver took me up and down mountain roads to Beirut on what I believe was the most frightening ride of my life. Imagine winding your way on narrow roads several thousand feet high, with no guard rails and countless hairpin curves. I was afraid to look down, for the drops seemed at least 1000 feet in many areas.

We finally arrived at the birthplace of both my father and mother. It was a touching occasion. I tried to realize the days over 60 years ago when my parents played as children in these humble surroundings. Now I, their son, had returned. I remember my stepfather returning to Lebanon 7 years ago. He recalls telling his mother before he left Lebanon in 1914 to keep his *ooud* (Lebanese guitar) in the closet as he expected to return in a year or so. Fifty years passed before he did return. He walked into his old stone homestead, opened the closet, and found his *ooud* still there, covered with a layer of dust but in excellent condition.

Amman And Refugees

And it was from my homeland Beirut that I flew into Amman, capital of Jordan. I wanted to view first-hand the refugee problem. While I had read of the plight of the refugees, I was not prepared for the utter hopelessness I was about to view.

The Pasha of Jordan made available to me his car and

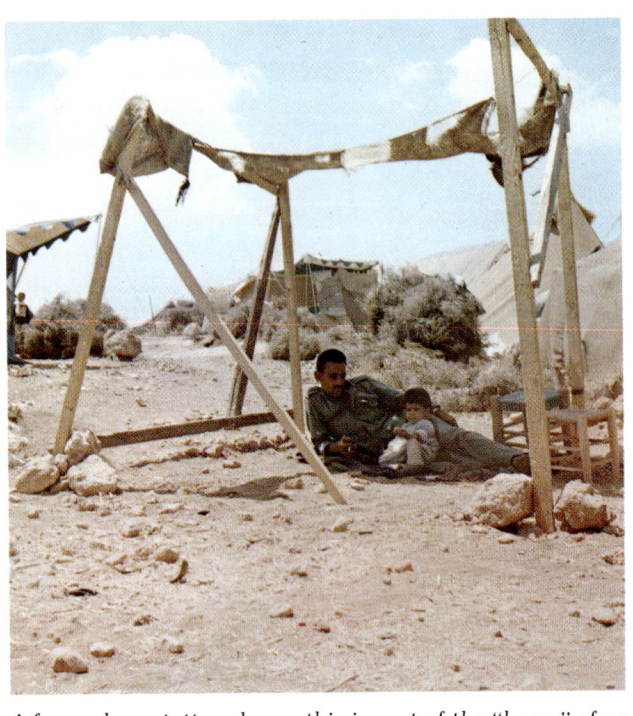

A few poles, a tattered rag...this is part of the "home" of an Arab father and his child.

driver for the day. UNRWA provided me with a representative to fill me in on the background. UNRWA is the United Nations Relief and Works Agency for Palestine Refugees in the Near East.

The UN Agency began work in May 1950; they provide the bulk of assistance to some 1 1/2 million refugees.

UNRWA defines a refugee as a person whose normal residence was Palestine for a minimum period of two years immediately before the conflict of 1948 and the recent war in 1967.

Most of the refugees are based in four host countries: Jordan, Gaza, Lebanon, and Syria. Of Jordan's population, as an example, about 50% are refugees and in the Gaza Strip, over 70%.

The problem is compounded by the fact that over 45,000 refugee babies are born annually.

Back in America we read that Israel has little concern for this problem. Israelites point to the fact that they, too, were refugees in World War II, but they quickly assimilated into the world and began new lives. Their contention is that the Arab states are using the refugee problem to win sympathy for their cause. There is much truth in this statement.

The Difference

It should be remembered, however, that many refugee Jews came from a heritage of industry and had basic valuable skills, while most Arab refugees were basically farmers, making their living from the land and using outdated methods. Many had very little schooling and no industrial skills. While the Jews have a heritage of creative industry, I found most Arabs did not possess these valuable talents or goals.

For over 90% of them the refugee camp is a dead end. There are no real opportunities. And basically few people in the world care about their plight.

On the other hand the Israel refugees of World War II received immense financial aid and the Israeli Government to this day receives about a million dollars a day in free aid.

As one Jordanian businessman told me, "Give me a million dollars a day and I, too, will make the desert blossom as a

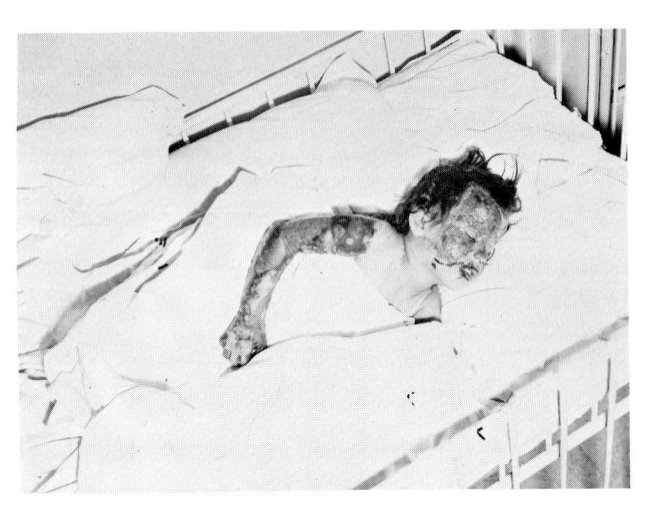

Today's intelligent society has given birth to devastating weapons of destruction...but how can you explain such "miracles" of war to this napalm burned Arab child?

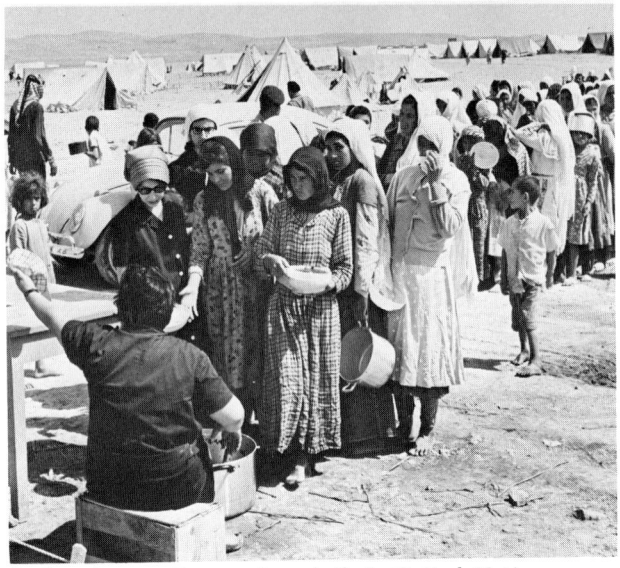

Arab refugees line up to get their United Nations emergency food rations at one of the emergency tent camps in East Jordan.

rose" (referring to the Scripture that prophesies that the Jewish people will make the Holy Land fertile again. Isaiah 35:1).

The work of UNRWA is to be commended, for they are doing the best they can under the circumstances and budget, but it is far from enough.

War resolves few problems. It does, however, create many problems. And presently the most pathetic of these is the refugees.

From A Home To A Hovel

We drove over the well-paved super highway from Amman (capital of Jordan) some 50 miles to Shuneh, a refugee camp just one month old with some 12,000 inhabitants. Imagine if you will, driving along a desert road and viewing on the horizon a city of tents nestled at the foot of a mountain.

From the macadam road we turned into a makeshift dirt road and I began an hour of baptism of red, sandy dust.

The sun was hot. Not a cloud was in the sky, and a modern American automobile driving into what appeared to be a tent town of Bible days made quite a contrast.

I was perhaps the first reporter to view this particular camp, and the first thing we had to do was meet the camp chief and secure permission to walk in the camp and take pictures.

I asked him how these people came here. He told me most had walked 50 to 100 miles from the West Bank of Jordan, leaving all their possessions as the Israeli Army forced them out.

"How did the Army force them out?" I inquired.

I was told that both subtle and external pressure was used. They were told to run for their lives; Israeli planes bombed their homes, and in some cases killed men, women and children, igniting terror in the natives and starting the mass exodus.

I walked around the camp interviewing and taking pictures. The camp leader cautioned me to be careful in photographing these people. Most are a proud people and are ashamed to have to live as they now do. I took photo of a young mother and a child—it so reminded me of Mary and the Christ child. I soon heard angry shouts in Arabic, a lan-

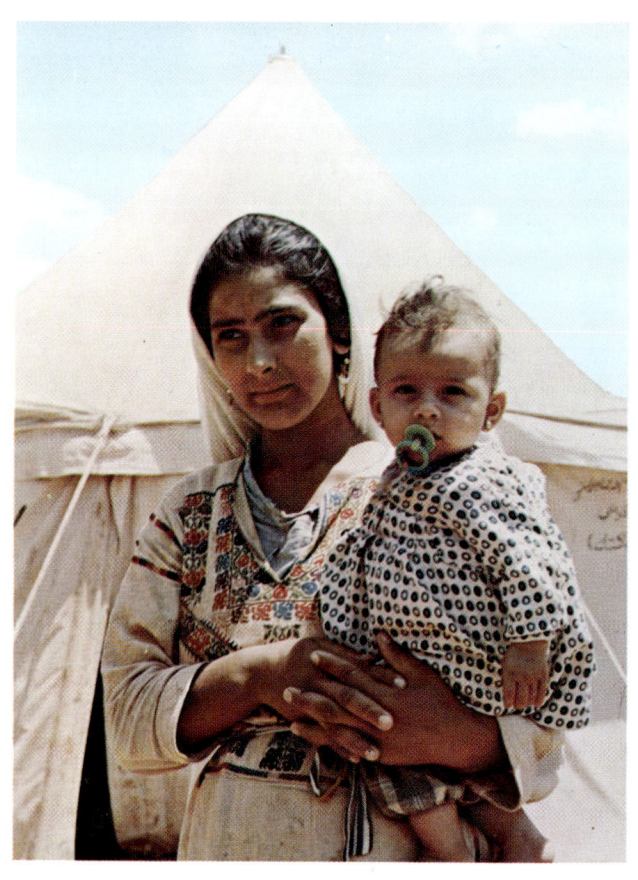

Arab mother in refugee camp near Amman, Jordan hopefully gazes towards Bethlehem from where she fled during 6-Day War.

guage I could not understand. A crowd of wild-eyed Arabs stormed around me and I was frightened.

My camp guide hurriedly shouted in Arabic to the crowd. Later I found that the Arabs had discovered I was an American and they resented my being there seeing them in their poverty.

The Camp Guide assured them I was of Arab descent and was their friend.

Behind The Flies . . . A Face!

The dust and flies are unimaginable unless you are actually there. Helpless little babies are huddled on the hot sand under the blinding sun, with running sores and their faces covered with swarming flies feasting on the sores, then crawling in the nostrils and mouth. A concerned mother brushes the flies away, but within 5 seconds they return.

It is hopeless. Everywhere there are flies.

Between every few tents is a mud wall about 4 feet high formed into a circle. This is their open air toilet. The flies use this as their homing base, and they cover the camp like a blanket, spreading disease.

In the midst of this tent city the only hint of civilization are the empty Sears, Roebuck boxes that contained the tents. One constantly sees women and children walking the mile to the spring, parading back balancing water cans on their heads.

And the children—they swarmed around me—excitedly jabbering away in Arabic, singing songs in praise of Nasser.

There is nothing for these people to do all day. They simply sit and wait. For some, their tent is just 4 poles with a weather-beaten rag stretched overhead. Others have tents donated by several countries, but these are unsuitable for the winter season, which is soon approaching when temperatures drop down to freezing.

Leaving All For Nothing At All

My guide discovered that his aunt and uncle were living in this camp and it was a joyous reunion. They insisted I sit down for Turkish coffee. I could not refuse.

They had been forced to flee their home in Jericho. They saw one of their friends, a 22-year old youth, shot and

I witnessed little Arab children with open sores that were covered with flies. Each spot on the child's face to the right...is a sore...and atop each sore, a fly! At that moment, I thanked God I was an American but my heart broke as I witnessed the suffering of my people. Again, how true the African proverb..."When the elephants go to war, it's the grass that gets trampled!"

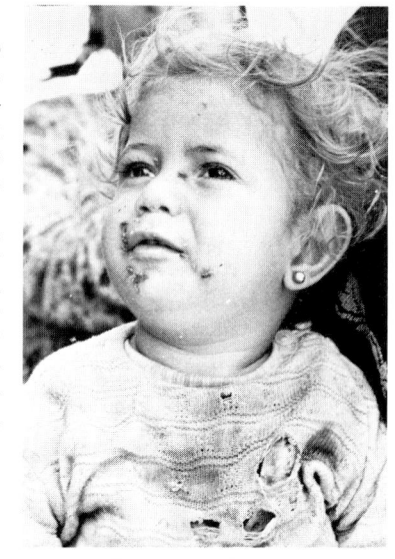

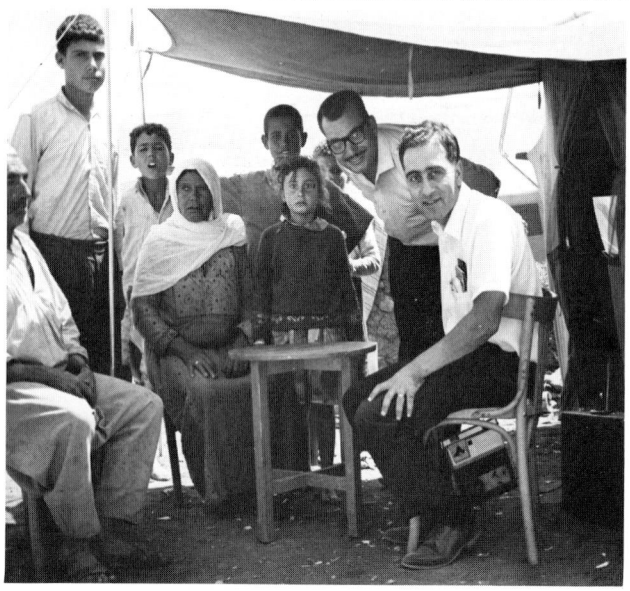

The Author sits down for a cup of Turkish coffee with a newly reunited family at a refugee camp near Amman, Jordan.

killed by an Israeli soldier because he did not want to leave his home. They saw the napalm bombs fall and told me of one husband who saw his wife horribly burned to death from a napalm bomb that made a direct hit on their car.

They had left a lifetime of possessions in their hometown of Jericho, formerly in Jordan but now a part of Israel. These possessions represented about $2500 in property and goods. This would be about $10,000 in American standards.

I drank Turkish coffee with them at their tent. I walked inside the tent to see what possessions they had brought with them. All I found were a couple pots and pans, a little coffee pot and four tiny coffee cups—from which they humbly served me. I had eaten in opulent restaurants, spotlessly clean. But now as the sand whipped across our faces—surrounded by hundreds of youngsters and by what appeared to be an equal number of flies determined to taste my coffee—somehow I felt at home. Here was humble truth unvarnished by the glittering selfishness of the world.

It was like a widow's mite. She had little to give the Lord but what she gave was her all.

And while I have never liked Turkish coffee, somehow it tasted good. And I wondered—in this world of war and suffering—is there no balm in Gilead? I watched the camp leader tenderly put his arm around a little waif . . . and I looked at the inquiring eyes of the children around me, who were dressed in tattered rags and browned by the constant dust, and I wished that every American could have the privilege of dining in my exclusive dining room.

I would not have traded this experience for anything.

And it is one I shall never forget.

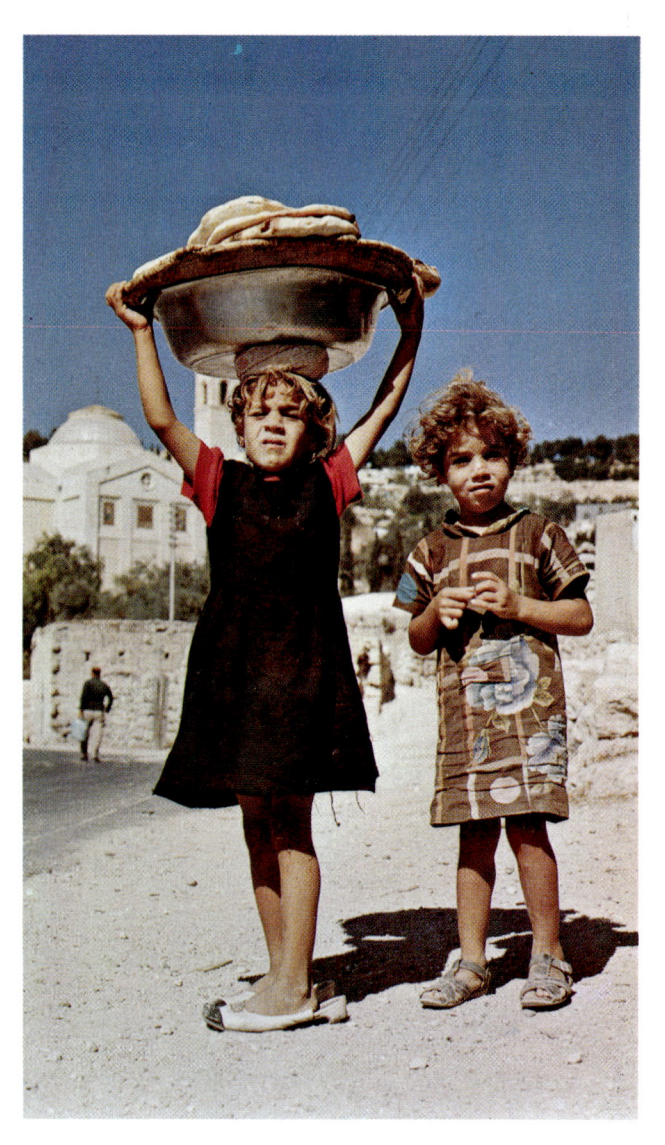

One of my favorite photographs. I took this picture in Bethany near Jerusalem. Two little Arab girls on their way home with freshly baked bread.

"THE DESERT SHALL BLOSSOM AS A ROSE"

War can be very inconvenient.

To reach Jerusalem from Amman one could not take the road for the 50 mile ride. The bridge had been bombed and traffic between Jordan and Israel was forbidden.

It was therefore necessary for me to fly from Amman, Jordan, to Nicosia, Cyprus (1 hour), spend a day and a half in Cyprus and then fly to Tel Aviv (1 hour).

While in Nicosia, I decided I wanted to visit some historic ruins on the coastline about 16 miles away. I was told that my Cypriot driver was not allowed to go through the Turkish settlement and that the drive to the coast would have to be 50 miles in a circuitous route. The day I was in Cyprus, a mother and child had been murdered in the eternal conflict of Turks (which represent 20% of the population) and the Cypriots.

My friends in Jordan had warned me that in Jerusalem I would find the areas occupied by the Jews filthy and that of the Arabs clean. I had learned by this time not to accept anything as fact until I saw it for myself.

As the plane circled to land in Tel Aviv, I was reading in the Cyprus Daily Mail newspaper some interesting news. The British were ousting a school principal for severely caning youngsters' bottoms while Israeli police were warn-

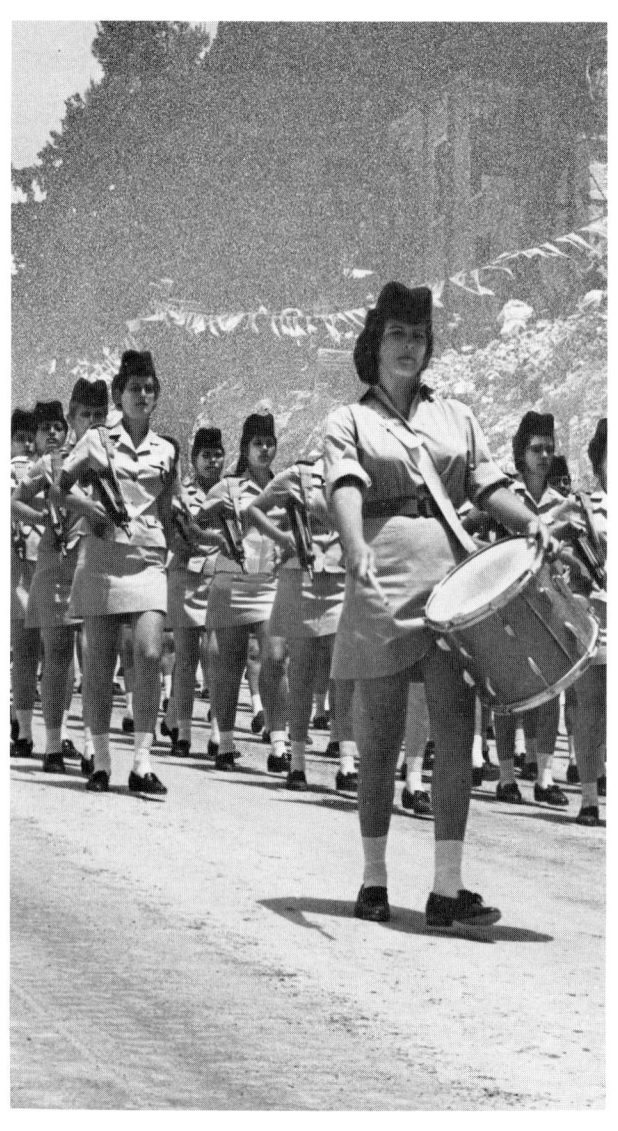

Mini-skirted Israeli women soldiers pass in review in parade shortly after 6-Day War.

ing Israeli girls not to wear mini-skirts in the Arab sector of Jerusalem because the Arabs (unused to such a sight) were pinching their bottoms.

It was late evening when I arrived in Tel Aviv, but even in the darkness one could notice the difference in the countryside, the efficiency of the customs inspectors at the airport, and the spirit of happiness among the people. This was quite a contrast from the barnlike structure air terminal of Saigon, with officials enmeshed in confusion and paper work, the poor airport facilities, the presence of soldiers in Amman, and the extensive checking of luggage in my own homeland. In Lebanon my cab driver had to stand against a wall and be searched by police before being allowed to enter the terminal.

Early the next morning I employed an English-speaking guide and we drive for about 1 1/2 hours to Jerusalem.

I had many times sung the anthem, "I walked today where Jesus walked," but the words were so familiar that they had lost their meaning. Now these words were to become a reality and I was overjoyed.

I soon experienced the great thrill the Israelis must have had to see Jerusalem back in their own hands. Although the UN had specifically given them the right of free travel from Tel Aviv to the Holy Shrines of Jerusalem, for 20 years they could not travel that road and for 20 years it was virtually a no man's land. Special convoys would travel, equipped with armor plate. But many brave drivers were killed by mines and sniper fire from Jordanian soldiers hidden along the roadside.

In memory of them, the Israeli Army left some of these tanks by the road, covered with a memorial wreath and markers as another symbol of Israel's continuing struggle for peace.

It's easy to tell when you reach the area that was occupied by Jordan before the six-day war.

The Contrast

On the Israeli side, the hills are an abundance of trees and shrubs; the plains have been made fertile with mechanized farm equipment tilling the soil. When you reach the pre-war Jordanian border, the hills are barren of vege-

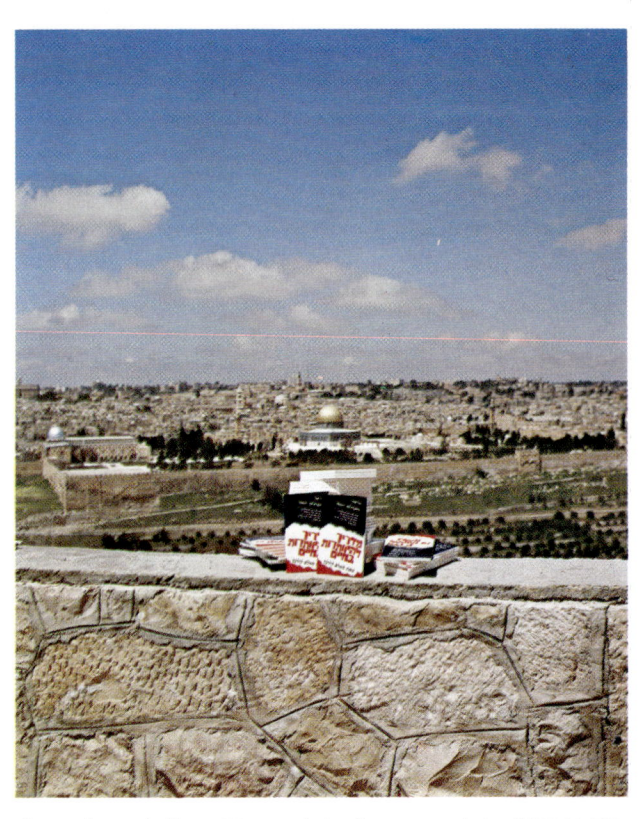

Jerusalem skyline. Pictured in foreground is GUIDE TO SURVIVAL in Hebrew...a book written by the Author. It has been said, "Ten portions of beauty descended to the world, Jerusalem acquired nine and the rest of the world, one."

tation, and the Arabs still use the primitive donkey for their farming.

Immediately after the six-day war, Israel paved an excellent road from Tel Aviv to Jerusalem, and within a month after the war they were expanding it into a modern four-lane highway. I was impressed at the speed and efficiency with which the Jewish nation operates. It was difficult for me to see evidence of the bombing as these damaged areas, for the most part, had been repaired and restored.

As we passed over the crest of a hill, there was Jerusalem in all its splendor—just as I had imagined it. Not a cloud in the sky—the valley dotted with stone structures similar to Bible times—a boy tending a herd of sheep—another riding a donkey. It was a superb setting.

Jerusalem—City Of Conflict

No city in history has been fought over so often—Jerusalem has endured 20 sieges. No city has been destroyed so often. Yes, no spot on earth has been won and lost by so many nations. A spring flowing out of the Kidron Valley provides a plentiful water supply, an excellent prize in this arid country.

Archeologists believe that Jerusalem was settled about 3000 B.C. by Bronze Age Canaanite tribesmen. When Abraham entered Palestine (Genesis 14) after his victories in Syria, he was greeted near the city by Melchizedek, King of Salem. Abraham prepared to sacrifice his son Isaac on a rock atop Jerusalem's Mount Moriah.

David captured Jerusalem from the Jebustites about 1000 B.C., and Solomon built a magnificent Temple to contain the Ark of the Covenant here.

To the Jews, Jerusalem represents "the place where Jehovah (the holy name for God) chose to dwell" (Deuteronomy 12:11). For Christians, it marks the spot where Christ was crucified and rose again; and for the Moslem, legend has it that Mohammed, borne from Mecca by a winged mare, ascended to Heaven from the site of Judaism's Temple. Christ, before He entered Jerusalem for the Last Supper, predicted the city's destruction declaring that its enemies would "not leave one stone upon another in you" (Matthew 24:2).

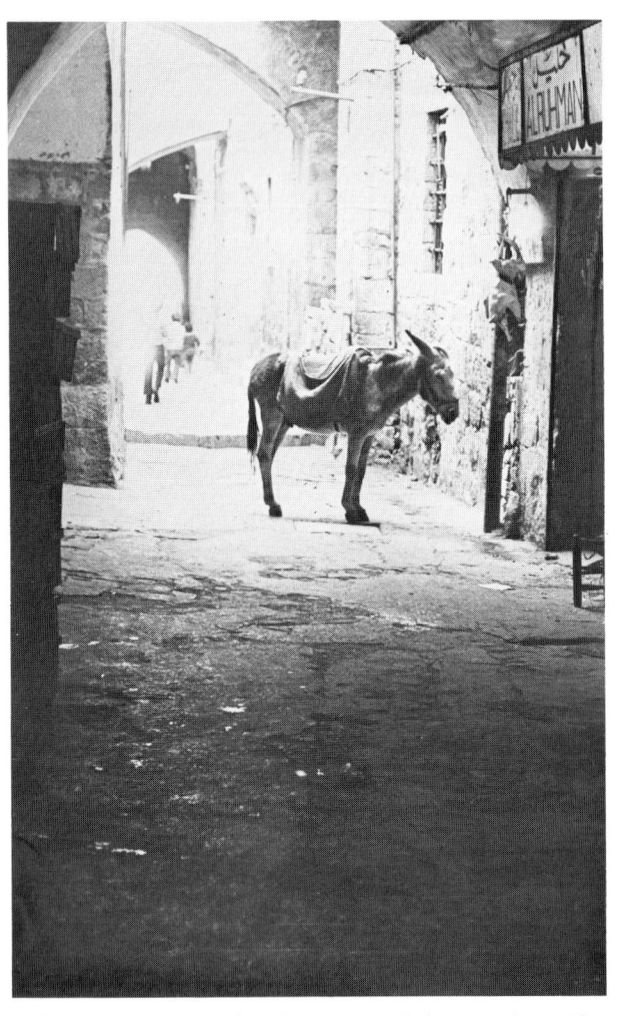

A donkey waits in a lonely courtyard in Jerusalem. This scene reminds us of Christ's Triumphal Entry into Jerusalem (Matthew 21:1-9). Peace will not come again to Jerusalem until Christ returns.

The Romans brought this destruction to pass in 70 A.D. The day I visited Jerusalem it was packed with tourists, most of them Israeli tourists coming for the first time to see their beloved shrines.

I watched in awe as men and women rushed to the Wailing Wall—men on the left side and women at the right. An Israeli soldier in uniform, with a sub-machine gun slung over his shoulder, was chanting at the wall a prayer for peace.

Everything was orderly and respectful.

Walking through the old city of Jerusalem, Arabs and Jews mingled freely.

The Tourist Plum

Israel had won a $35 million Tourist plum in Jerusalem that was bound to double in a short time.

Where Jordan did not permit free access, Israel welcomed everybody. Where Jordan did not allow photography, Israel permitted photos anywhere. Where Jordan charged entrance fees to see the Holy City, Israel charged nothing.

The capture of Jerusalem by Israel can be counted a real blessing for the Free World, for Jerusalem is now truly a city accessible to all, even the Arabs, and each religion at last has free access to their holy shrines.

In talking to Mr. Yigal Allon, the Minister of Labor of Israel, he said that Israel will never give up its annexation of Jerusalem. For the first time in history, they can flock to the wailing wall, the only authentic remnant of Solomon's Temple, representing the most sacred part of Jewry.

From Jerusalem I took a 15 minute drive to Bethlehem. Here, too, Jews were in lines a block long to see Rachael's tomb.

But they also surprisingly showed an equal interest in viewing the place where Christ was born.

At Bethlehem I visited a hospital for crippled children. Ninety per cent of these children were crippled by polio under Jordanian rule. I saw a baby 12 months old with deep burns covering the body. The old custom was to apply a hot coal to a nerve and cause such pain it would supposedly drive the illness out.

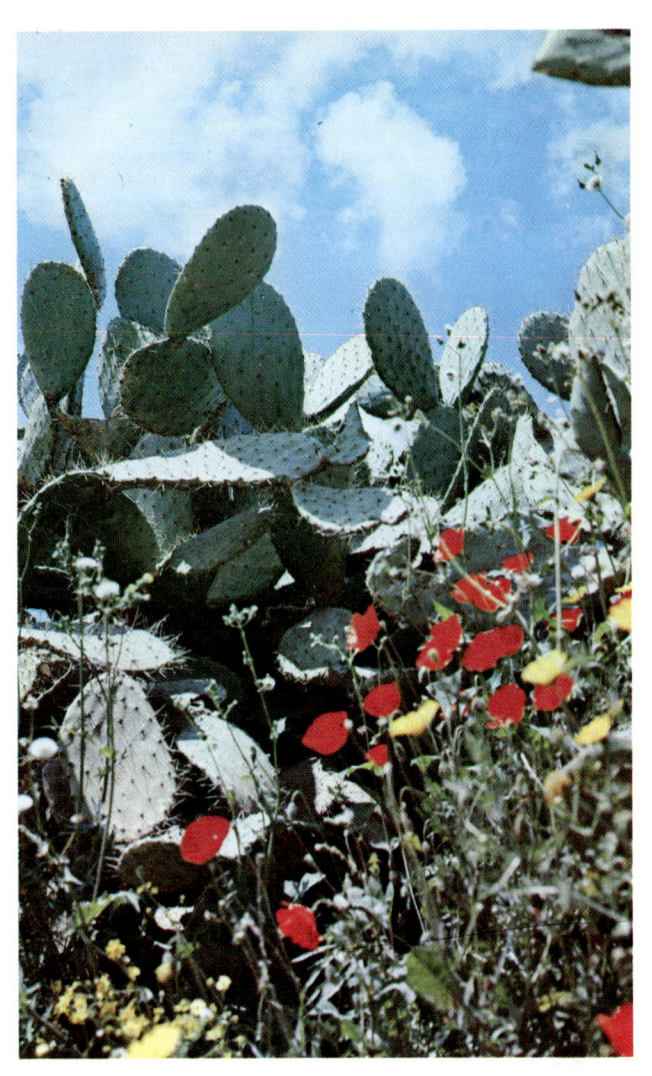

This beautiful photograph taken in Israel graphically portrays the people of Israel. Sabra is the fruit of cactus plant, prickly outside, sweet inside. Sabra is now a term to designate Israeli-born Jews. Israel's future will have the thorns of adversity until Christ reigns in the 1000-year Millennium Period.

Vaccines for polio have been in existence for over a decade; mechanized equipment, for at least 35 years. And yet I found my own people—the Arabs—sometimes painfully slow in their progress.

My own face-to-face examination of both Arab countries and Israel found many on each side sincerely wanting peace.

Coming to Israel from the refugee camps was truly like coming to God's Promised Land.

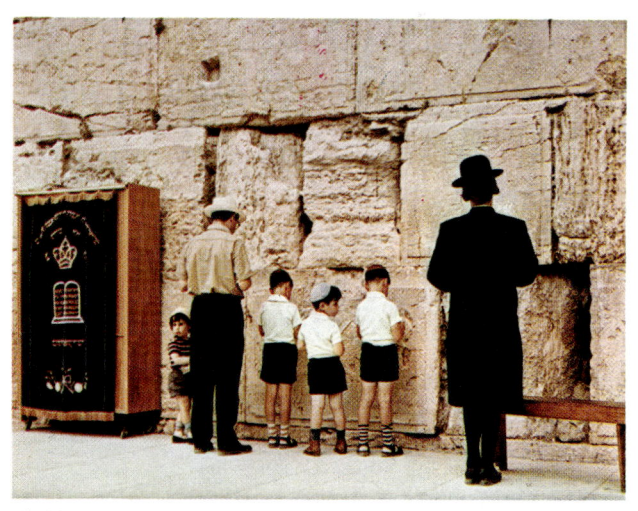

Children stand with their father at the Wailing Wall, unaware of the tragedy that surrounds them.

Waiting for something to eat, these are two of the thousands of innocent victims of the war in the Middle East.

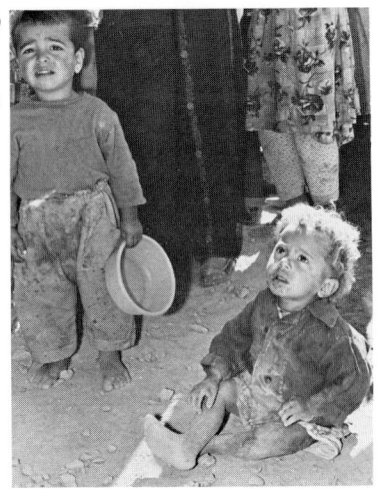

THIS WAS PALESTINE

The words "Palestine" and "Palestinian" are often in the Middle East news these days. Here, briefly, is their meaning:

Palestine, the area that was long under Turkish rule ...then under British mandate before Israel was created in 1948...no longer exists as an entity. In general, it means Holy Land. The word PALESTINE comes from the Greek for Philistia, home of the ancient Philistines. The area has been split between Israel and Jordan since 1948.

Palestinians in general are the Arabs who lived in Palestine under the British mandate, or those who are descended from these people.

About 800,000 of these left when Israel was created or fled during the Arab-Israeli war that began then. Many of them and their descendants still occupy refugee camps, mostly in Jordan or the Gaza Strip along the Mediterranean.

HELLO, MR. PRESIDENT!

The warm sun of Tel Aviv was bidding me stay, but my heart strings were tugging me home.

Riding in the cab to the airport the radio was blarring
> "Give me land, lots of land
>   'neath the starry sky above,
> Don't fence me in."

And I was saying goodbye to a happy Israeli people who had seen their fondest dreams come true in just six short days.

My trip was now ending. It was hard to believe that in just 27 days I had visited hot spots in 10 different countries.

Prior to my trip, many had questioned the advisability of it. "How could you," they said, "expect to discover the real issues and analyze the problems in just a day or two in each country? You must spend many months in each area."

And for a while I believed them.

But in each country I made it a point to pick the brains of the knowledgeable people of that country—from the politician or military leader (whose remarks I took with a grain of salt) and more important the man-in-the-street, the humble native, the missionary, the businessman, the desk

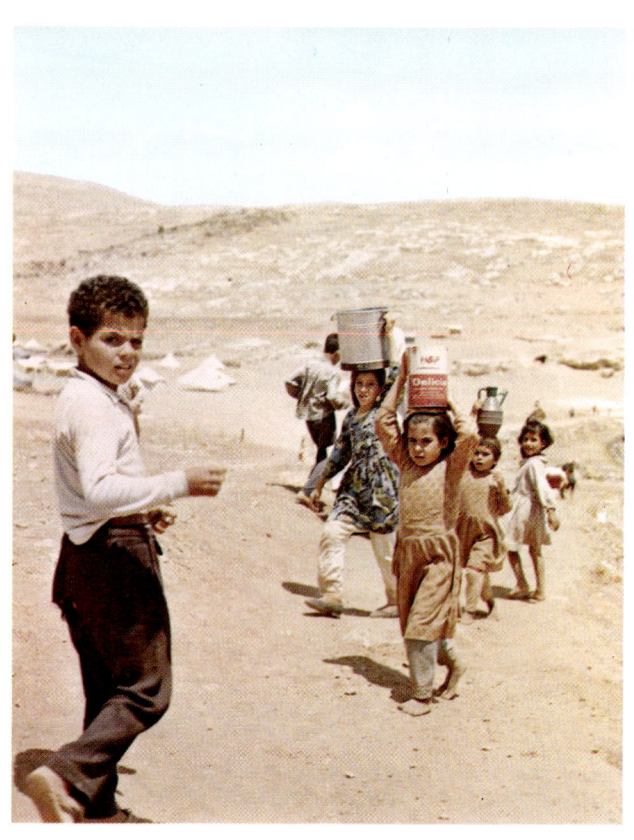

Refugee children at camp in Amman, Jordan, carry water back to their tents.

clerk and where necessary, people who were present when certain war crises took place.

I found a real advantage in this whirlwind 27 day tour of the major hot spots of the world. I was able to cover all these areas in a short enough time to develop a true perspective of the present world situation. This would not be true had I spent a month or two in each country.

Truth vs. Fiction

As an example, the Lebanese said that the refugees were well taken care of by the Jordan government. The next day I was in Jordan and found just the opposite. The Jordanians told me that the streets occupied by the Jews in Jerusalem were filthy. Two days later I was in Jerusalem and found quite the contrary.

Other sources had told me the napalm bombing of Jordanians was insignificant. I witnessed the tragic consequences of horribly burnt bodies and thought otherwise.

A prominent Israeli leader in government told me that the Arabs were not forced to leave their homes when the Israeli Army occupied the land. The refugees in Jordan told me they were. The next day I visited Bethlehem and, in interviewing reliable witnesses, found that the fact was that Israeli sound trucks had entered Bethlehem, instructing Arabs to get out and to leave by an old road.

Likewise, in an interview with General Westmoreland, we newsmen asked the General what accomplishments the U.S. had made in Vietnam in the last two years. After a moment of hesitation he stated, "Roads have been made secure."

The next few days I travelled throughout Vietnam interviewing soldiers in their field. Their consensus—no road in Vietnam was secure. Heavy enemy action in and around Saigon, and attempts to blow up the Rex Hotel where I daily attended press conferences made this fact even more evident.

These are some of the areas of analysis that could best be made by a quick, efficient whirlwind reporting tour.

And within 27 days the result of all this data enabled me to synthesize the dross and find the real problems of the

VIETNAM PEACE
TOLL OF A COSTLY WAR

IN LIVES...

American servicemen killed in action:

World War II 291,557
Civil War
  (North and South) 234,938
World War I 53,402
Vietnam war **45,937**
Korean War 33,629
Revolutionary War 4,435
War of 1812 2,260
Mexican War 1,733
Spanish-American War 385

IN WOUNDED...

American servicemen wounded in action:

World War II 670,846
Civil War
  (North and South) 382,000
Vietnam war **303,622**
World War I 204,002
Korean War 103,284
Revolutionary War 6,188
War of 1812 4,505
Mexican War 4,152
Spanish-American War 1,662

IN LENGTH...

Vietnam war   **11 years, 1 month**
Revolutionary
  War .... 7 years, 8 months
Civil War .... 4 years
World War II .. 3 years, 8 months
Korean War .... 3 years
War of 1812 .. 2 years, 8 months
Mexican War .. 1 year, 9 months
World War I .. 1 year, 7 months
Spanish-American
  War .... 4 months

IN DOLLARS...

                        Military Spending

World War II .... $341 billion
Vietnam war .... **$140 billion**
Korean War .... $54 billion
World War I .... $25.7 billion
Civil War
  (North only) .... $4 billion
Spanish-American
  War .... $576 million
Mexican War ...... $166 million
War of 1812 .... $134 million
Revolutionary War ... $75 million

...AND ALSO COSTLY IN AIR LOSSES

Aircraft lost in Vietnam war—

	Airplanes	Helicopters
IN COMBAT	1,646	2,280
IN ACCIDENTS, OTHER NONHOSTILE CAUSES	2,098	2,588
TOTAL	**3,744**	**4,868**

world, its present condition, and the possible solutions to world peace.

And the picture is not a bright one.

America has come of age. And blind patriotism should make way for not only responsible citizenship, but responsible leadership.

I remember standing in the desert of the Middle East and viewing the ruins of what were once opulent, flourishing Roman cities. Now they were but crumbled stones and decay—their only company is the desert lizard and the flowering thorn.

I do not want my country, the United States, with such a wonderful heritage, to be the recipient of a like demise.

And yet we seem headed for such self-destruction at a jet-speed rate.

Living For Today

Americans are excercising freedom at the expenses of sanity. So called leaders of society uphold what in my opinion is obscenity, both in leadership and readership. Our laws are lax in both directions. We seem content to ride the roller coaster of "Eat, drink and be merry."

And yet our government forbids prayers in public schools.

America has made mistakes. It should be adult enough not only to admit them but rectify them.

We justified sending our boys 10,000 miles away by saying we must "contain communism." Sometimes we must also give some serious thought to "containing Democracy" . . . for in our political expediency to fight a war 10,000 miles away, the Cuban well-spring of Communism ferments right within our gates and Congress has difficulty in pushing through $40 million to fight rats in slum areas in our own country.

In my interviews throughout the world people were disturbed that American leaders deal lightly with corruption in their own ranks and speak with a "forked tongue."

In Japan I found people deeply concerned about seeking solutions for peace. People in that country were still dying from the A-bomb blasts of over 20 years ago.

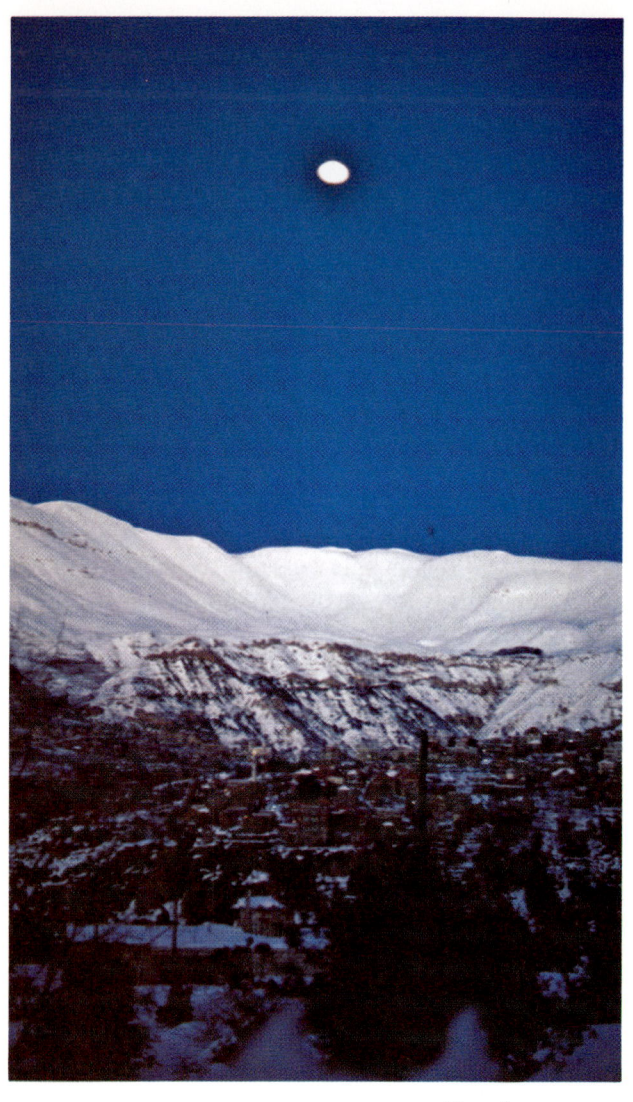

Photo by Larry Rink

Lebanon, a country of unexcelled beauty. Pictured is a winter scene at the village of Kahlil Gibran (1883-1931), poet, philosopher and artist.

In Vietnam I found a country divided in spirit and in purpose. Over 50,000 Americans have died on Vietnamese soil. Historians, in my opinion, should report our entry and conduct of the Vietnam War as America's greatest blunder.

If there could be any commitment for involvement it would have been in the Israeli struggle for survival. Fortunately for the United States, the Israeli had enough sense of national pride, sacrifice, and unity of purpose to take care of his own problems.

Even Jordan, receiving some $35 million a year from the U.S., is sincerely guiding its economy so it won't have to lean on American aid.

Time To Grow Up

Some Arab leaders are spending too much time spewing hate at the expense of backward living conditions of their people. While they claim they will never do so, they must recognize Israel as a sovereign and equal country. It is my hope that responsible Arab leaders have the courage to be honest with their people rather than sacrifice right for personal political expediency.

Israel, too has made mistakes but they show a sincere willingness to cooperate with their Arab neighbors, economically and socially. They have a sense of pride and accomplishment. They are a new-born babe in the Middle East, but in some areas they are years ahead in progress over their Arab neighbors. And it's about time the Arabs wake up to the facts of life.

This trip was a real eye-opener for me, for I learned many things one does not read in the newspapers back home.

Being of Arab parentage, my purpose in going to the Middle East was originally to present the Arab side of the story. But after seeing both sides of the issue first hand, I had to honestly admit that some Arab leaders were doing a disservice to their countrymen.

Seeking solutions to peace was the main purpose of my trip. There were not going to be any hard and fast answers.

But one thing I found certain—war was not going to resolve problems. Today the problems are Vietnam and the Middle East. Tomorrow they may be Cuba and the Congo.

NEW YORK, SUNDAY, MAY 19, 1974

INDIA BECOMES 6TH NATION TO SET OFF NUCLEAR DEVICE

ANNOUNCES BLAST

Soviets Mobilized for Mideast
7 Divisions Readied Last October, Reports Say

By MURREY MARDER
Washington Post Service

WASHINGTON — The Soviet Union is reported boasting that it mobilized seven Russian divisions to fight for Egypt last October.

The published reports, now circulating across the Middle East, cannot be independently authenticated. If verified, would be the first Soviet admission of what the United States charged was happening, resulting in the American global military alert the night of Oct...

openly moving closer to the United States, to the dismay of the Soviet Union.

The Soviet Union, in turn, is appealing over the head of Egyptian President Anwar Sadat to try to demonstrate that it has been loyal to Arab nationalism.

Much of what is being said on both sides "has the ring of authenticity to it" and basically "is credible" when compared with information known to American intelligence, U. S. sources said Wednesday.

to "a number of Egyptian official and political personalities."

Vinogradov is now the Soviet ambassador in Geneva for the Middle East peace talks.

The As Safir article came to the attention of officials in Washington when it was reprinted next day by the Beirut newspaper An Nida, which American sources say is a Communist organ supporting the line of the Soviet Communist Party. An Nida

during the October war," which began on Oct. 6, 1973.

Its account of the October alert attributed to Vinogradov is as follows:

"In the early hours of 20 October, at exactly 0300, President Sadat contacted me and asked me to convey an urgent message on the situation to Brezhnev (Soviet Communist Party chief Leonid I. Brezhnev) and ask him to intervene to achieve an immediate cease-fire.

"I contacted Moscow. The director of the office informed me that Comrade Brezhnev had gone to bed only one hour before and that he could not wake him up. I asked him to wake him up on my responsibility. I informed Brezhnev of the situation as explained by President Sadat and his request.

"The Soviet leaders immediately issued a decision for a partial alert of the Soviet forces. Seven Soviet military...

Pentagon Wastes $200 Million On More Nerve Gas When Stockpiles Are Enough to Kill Entire World

The U.S. Army is literally throwing away $200 million to develop a new strain of nerve gas while spending $300 million to destroy the lot it already has.

Despite possessing enough chemical warfare stockpile to wipe out the entire world population, the Pentagon claims that supply is not enough.

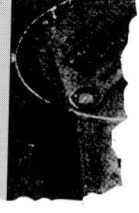

Gas storage areas near many major U.S. cities simply are not safe and present an extreme danger to those living nearby, Department of Defense spokesmen admit.

The new gas the Pentagon seeks will hopefully eliminate threat of a major catastrophe from enemy attack. The new system will consist of two components, each comparatively harmless until combined with the other.

These components will be stored separately, only to be brought together when needed for an attack, Pentagon officials claim.

This move appears beneficial to the American public, but is best one more...

By WILLIAM BARNHILL
and MARTY GUNTHER

development, it's common knowledge that one of the compounds resembles household insecticides, while the other is a simple alcohol compound that can be purchased commercially.

When combined, only one tiny drop — the size of the period at the end of this sentence — is enough to kill a human in minutes.

IF THIS formula fell into the hands of any fanatical terrorist group, it would provide...

proposed weapons which have very questionable utility, this is the only one which even the Pentagon admits has very little military usefulness.

"AND YET — in the very epitome of ill-conceived judgment — the Nixon Administration is willing to spend more than $200 million on a weapon that poses a much more serious threat to the civilian population in this country than to any potential enemy," Abourezk charged.

"If the prime reason for developing these binary weapons is the one the Army claims — to reduce the hazards inherent in present stockpiles of nerve agents — the same objective can be achieved by better, safer and cheaper means:

"Simply abolish the stockpiles in their entirety.

---

26 *The Evening Bulletin* Friday, March 29, 1974

Future Food May Be Bacteria That Feed on Trash

Baton Rouge, La. — (UPI) — With the help of some hungry bacteria Dr. Clayton Callihan and his colleagues hope to end the mountains of trash in the world.

Callihan is a member of a Louisiana State University research team working on a project to harvest protein-rich bacteria grown on a cellulose waste solution.

"We could almost feed the world with the protein available in the United States," said Callihan, a chemical engineering professor.

He uncorked a jar of brown crumbs and sprinkled out a few grains of what may be the food of the future.

The crumbs taste like bland crackers, but Callihan said that by adding the proper flavor a cook may one day be able to turn out anything from steak to bacon and eggs.

Planned

LSU recently entered into a contract with Bechtel International, a San Francisco engineering firm, to build a $18 million demonstration plant to begin manufacturing the food

for use as a protein supplement for animals.

By the end of the decade Callihan hopes it may be used for human diets as an inexpensive source of high protein.

"Steak is only about 22 percent protein. Our bugs run almost 80 percent protein," said Callihan.

The process developed by

Callihan, Dr. Vadake P. Srivanaven and several other LSU scientists starts with cellulose wastes such as paper, leaves, trees, sawdust or sugar cane stalks.

"Our microorganisms don't seem to care much where the cellulose comes from, they'll eat it regardless," said Callihan. "The only preference

we've really found is in computer printout paper. They really like that.

"We grow bugs on cellulose. We feed them the cellulose, they eat it, and when they get big enough we harvest them."

The cellulose is first ground, then cleaned in a special solution, heated and then washed again. It is put in fermenters...

These problems are generated by greed and personal ambition. They are watered by distrust and lack of communication. And the fruit they bear is one of tanks and arms and planes and bombs and world chaos.

The United States should exercise just as much ingenuity and money to seek and work out solutions for peace as it so recklessly enters its instruments for war at the drop of the proverbial "commitment" hat.

Twenty-seven days ago I said "Goodbye Mr. President" when he would not grant me a personal interview to "come now let us reason together."

Now 27 days later, I return to the country I love and say "Hello, Mr. President." The answer to world problems is a deep abiding faith in God that will allow our actions to be controlled by the tenets of this faith.

Then, Mr. President, while you so often paraphrase
    "Come now let us reason together,"
you can continue the balance of that verse which ends
    "though your sins be as scarlet,
    they shall be as white as snow."

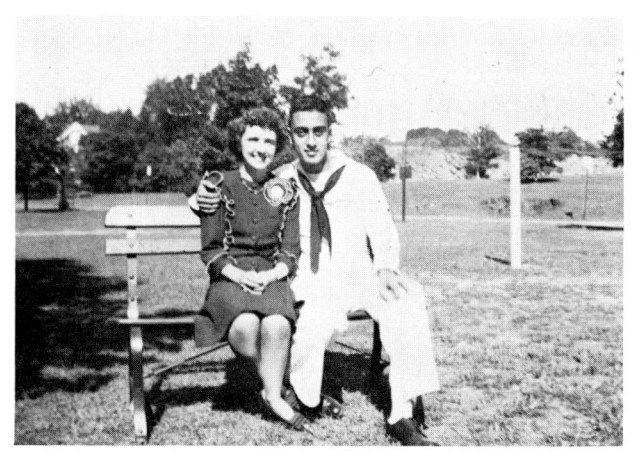

True love. I first met Mary Stevenson in 1943. Our first date was January 18, 1944...the day I was drafted. That night I took the midnight train to Sampson, New York for Navy boot camp. This photo was taken in Elkins Park...a suburb of Philadelphia, in 1944 during a weekend leave. Mary Stevenson became Mary Kirban!

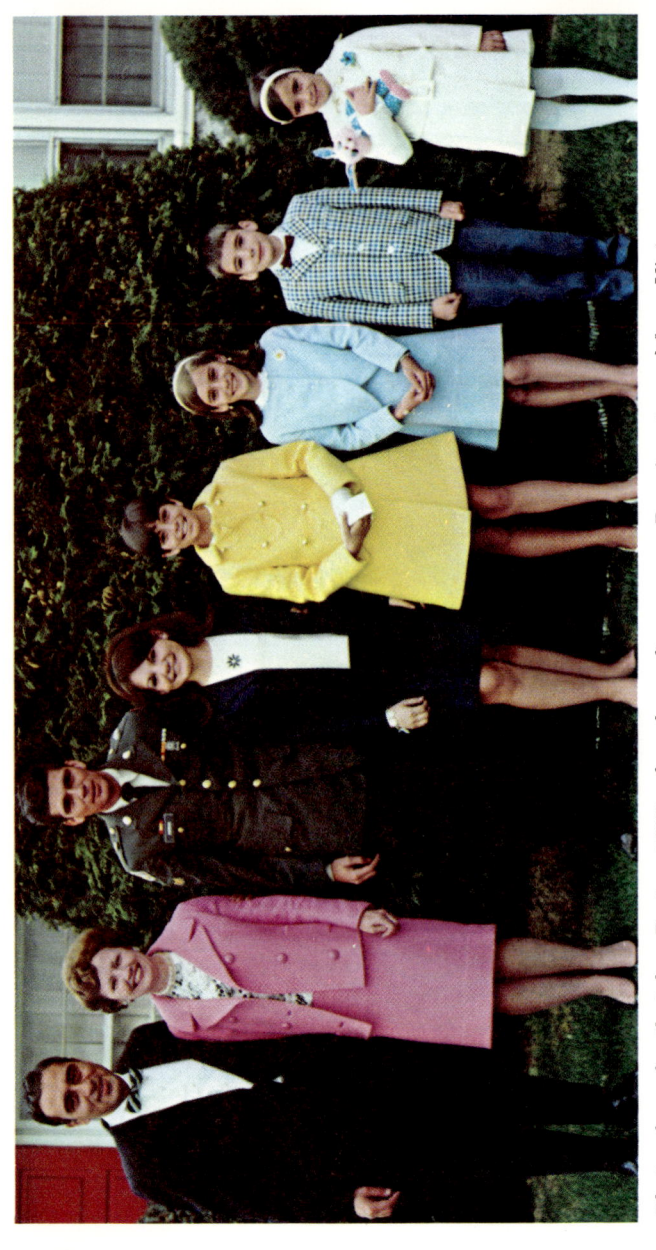

Photo of our family taken Easter, 1968 a few days after our son Dennis returned from Vietnam. The author; my dear wife, Mary; Dennis and his wife, Eileen; Doreen, Diane, Duane and our youngest, Dawn.

IN CONCLUSION

Can America make a mistake?

While many did not agree with Governor Rommey one must give him credit for having had the courage to admit he erred in his Vietnam policy.

For making this statement he was held up to ridicule by many American leaders.

Many Americans hold the view that America makes no mistakes — and if it does — should not admit them for danger of losing face.

In my opinion this policy can only lead to disaster. It takes far greater courage and patriotism to admit an error and then seek to correct it . . . even though it may not be the popular choice.

Girard College . . . Responsibility

At Girard College I learned that with freedom comes responsibility. Responsible citizenship must rise above the flag wavers and the peace marchers and constructively build a better America.

Many people seem to forget first that America was a nation founded under God . . . and this neglect may be the root of all our rapidly multiplying problems.

Could it be that we are seeing a re-enactment of the era that saw the spiritual, moral and physical decay of the Roman empire?

Nixon Vows He'll 'Never Give Up'

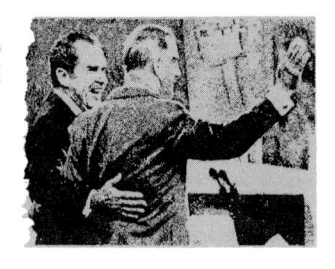

The New York Times

VOL.CXXIII...No 42,512 — NEW YORK, THURSDAY, JUNE 13, 1974 —

Cheering Cairo Throngs Greet Nixon
Sadat Hails His Guest as Man of Peace

CAPITAL RALLYING ROUND KISSINGER
VINDICATION ASKED
Judge Decides Ehrlichman Can Be Tried With Others
Gesell Says White House Eases Claim of Executive Privilege — Hints Trial

The Cincinnati Post

Friday evening, June 14, 1974 — Cincinnati's Largest Daily Newspaper — Weather: Partly cloudy, warmer

U.S. TO SELL A-DATA TO EGYPT

NIXON PROMISES LONG-TERM HELP FOR THE ISRAELIS

Pledges Arms and Economic Aid — Bids New Cabinet Take Risks for Peace

NUCLEAR PACT PLANNED

Joint Statement Says U.S. Will Negotiate Accord on Atomic Cooperation

---

THURSDAY, JULY 4, 1974

NIXON, BREZHNEV DELAY KEY CURBS ON ARMS TILL '85

To Seek New Interim Pact on Offensive Missiles as Summit Effort Fails

MOSCOW MEETING ENDS

Kissinger Hints Military on Both Sides Still Oppose Permanent Limitations

Prayer has been outlawed in public schools, the loyalty oath has been termed unconstitutional by the U.S. Supreme Court, and more legal rulings encourage the rampage of pornography.

It would not surprise me that "America, America, God shed His grace on thee" be changed to "America, America, Our grace is shed on thee."

Some leaders recklessly throw around the term Communism or Communist-inspired on most anything that disagrees with their particular point of view.

Our involvement in Vietnam was based on the assumption that we must prevent the spread of Communism—and we must admit that Communism is indeed evil. One aspect, however, of Communism is that the destiny of many is controlled by the hands of a few. Could this same pattern be the direction into which America is now drifting? Many Americans are concerned and many Congressmen are embarrassed by the fact that perhaps unwittingly they have permitted the President of the United States an unusually wide range of personal power to commit an entire nation to war.

Towards Central Control

Can it be that a nation which was founded on wide representation now find itself spiralling towards more individual central control? And if so, can this be the Democracy that George Washington, Thomas Jefferson and Benjamin Franklin had in mind?

What has happened to the Monroe Doctrine? After the Bay of Pigs we secretly guaranteed not to molest Fidel Castro if the Soviets took the missiles out. Our Navy, Air Force and Coast Guard enforce a "blockade" around Red Cuba, not to quarantine and contain Castro but to protect his Communist rule from interference.

While on the other hand our men and money were sent to Vietnam to molest and contain the Viet Cong.

Yet we arrested any Cuban freedom fighter en route to their tortured homeland, impound their boats and private automobiles . . . and allow Russia to become Castro's paymaster—to the tune of about $400 million a year.

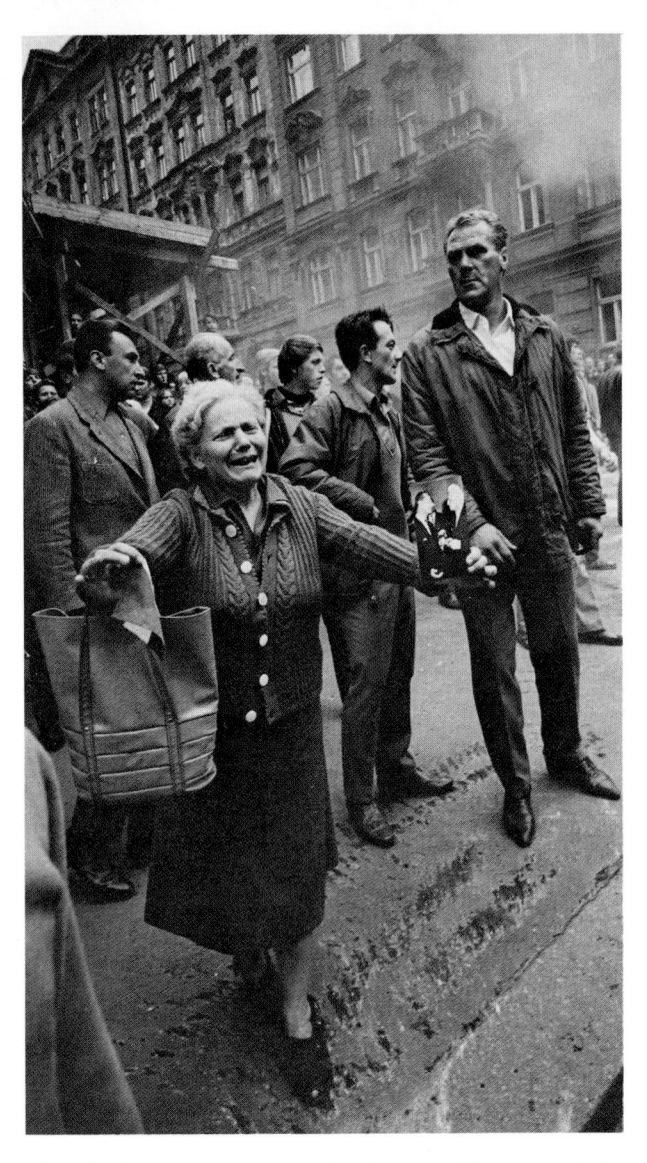

A Czechoslovakian woman cries in anguish as she holds photo of her country's leaders in defiance of invading Russian troops.

Nor can we forget a united Hungary that cried for help in its fight for freedom . . . only to receive a deaf ear from the United States and our inaction as we watched Russia build the Berlin wall. Here were clear clarion calls for freedom. Vietnam is not!

And with a deficit some say is approaching $75 billion, is America on the road to further taxation and less representation?

I would gladly work for my country for $1 a year on the "Little Nobody Committee" . . . a Committee I would suggest be created to find ways to save money in Government. Too many well-known personages make investigative trips, but far too often only reach the top brass—generals, admirals and high echelon leaders—returning with only what the leaders want them to hear. "Little Nobodys" could do some grass roots investigating and, in my opinion, show the Government how millions of dollars can be saved the U.S. taxpayer every month! This, I feel, is one step toward responsible citizenship.

Then, too, it might be well for all of us to remember the 4th stanza of THE STAR SPANGLED BANNER . . . which ends

> Blest with vict'ry and peace,
>   may the Heav'n-rescued land
> Praise the Pow'r that hath made
>   and preserved us a nation!
>
> Then conquer we must,
>   when our cause it is just;
> And this be our motto:
>   "In God is our trust!"
>
> And the star-spangled banner
>   in triumph shall wave
> O'er the land of the free,
>   and the home of the brave.

ABOUT THE AUTHOR

Salem Kirban is a graduate of Girard College and received his Bachelor of Science at Temple University in Philadelphia.

He and his wife Mary became more vitally concerned over world conditions when their son, Dennis, enlisted in the Army. The below Ad first appeared in The WASHINGTON POST prior to Salem Kirban's Round the World reporting trip.

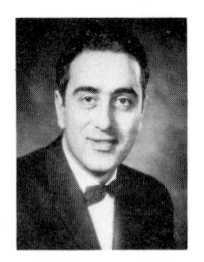

An Open Letter to President Johnson

GOODBYE MR. PRESIDENT...

On March 25th I wrote you requesting a personal interview. My son was sent to Viet Nam and as a concerned father I wanted more information on our commitment to that country.

I was aware of your phrase, "Come now, let us reason together"* and wanted to do just that. However, your office wrote that your schedule would not permit a personal interview. So I decided to do the next best thing—fly to Viet Nam, Israel, Egypt, Jordan and Russia and prepare a Citizen's Report on the Search for Peace.

I believe every American Citizen has first a duty to his country, and because of this privileged citizenship, also a responsibility to the world.

Now, as a citizen, under your leadership, I embark on my own Private Citizen Fact Finding mission around the world. I am sponsored by no one. I can report the facts accurately as I see them...and without bias.

I will be leaving from Philadelphia's International Airport this Sunday, July 16th at 6:15 P.M. on United Air Lines. I would consider it a real honor to have you send me off.

SALEM KIRBAN

P.S. If you can't make it this Sunday, will you grant me the privilege of personally presenting you with my Private Citizen Report on World Conditions...upon my return in Mid-August?

P.P.S. *This phrase is a part of a favorite Bible verse of mine... but you've only been quoting the first half of it. The second half offers the world's only hope for enduring peace. It's found in Isaiah 1:18.

SEQUEL

It has been seven years now since I made that unforgettable trip around the world in search for peace.

Seven years ago I wrote that the war in Vietnam was a mistake.

The United States frequently spent more in one month (close to $3 billion) than Russia spent through its counterpart, North Vietnam, in one year! For Russia it was a good investment...spending some $2-3 billion a **year** to force us to spend that amount **each month!**

The difference: We were personally involved with men and material. Some of our bombing strikes cost the U.S. as much as $15 million a day!

Today, I feel that many more now realize that this war only served as a means of further weakening the power of the United States.

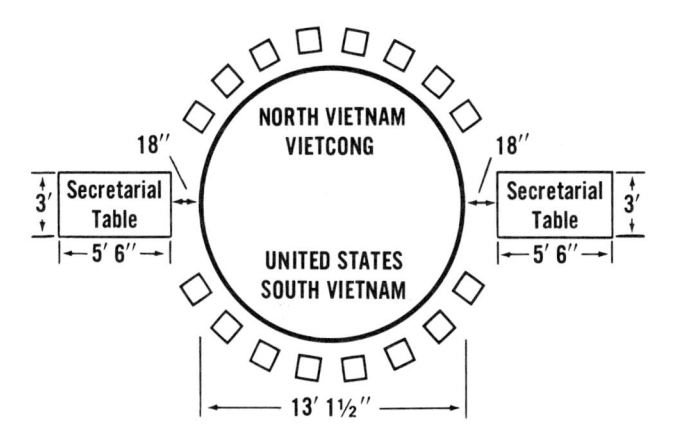

It took some four years of negotiation at Paris before a semblance of peace was realized. One man wrote:

> It is a sad bit of irony that man is able to construct a vehicle that can convey him safely on a 500,000-mile trip through space, but unable to design a table that will accommodate him so that he might embark upon a journey to peace!

At the peace negotiations, during the Vietnam War, the

145

Wife Sues for Divorce From Returned POW

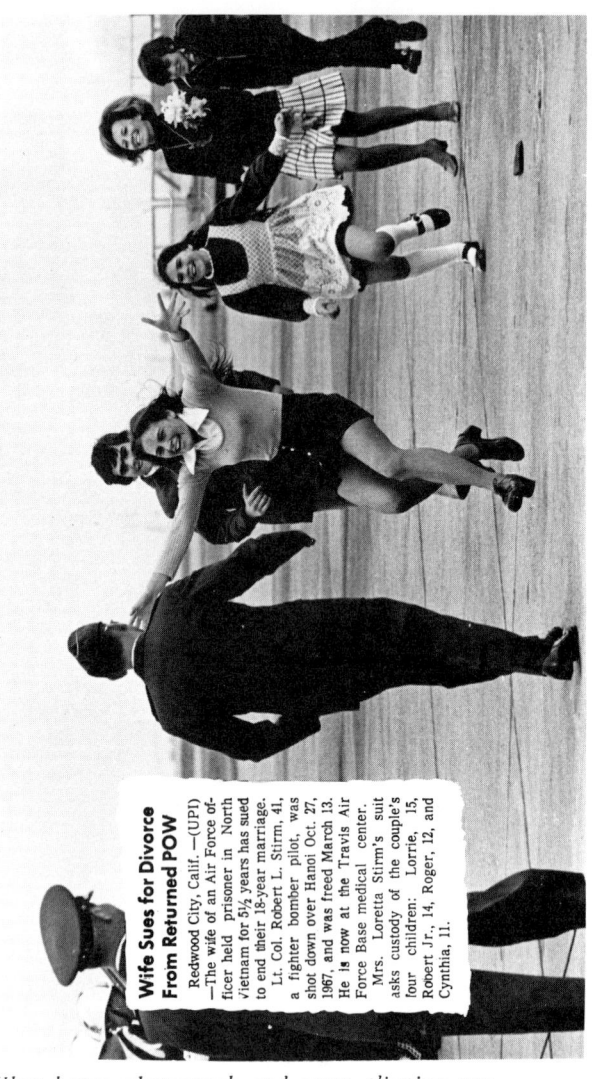

Redwood City, Calif. —(UPI) —The wife of an Air Force officer held prisoner in North Vietnam for 5½ years has sued to end their 18-year marriage.

Lt. Col. Robert L. Stirm, 41, a fighter bomber pilot, was shot down over Hanoi Oct. 27, 1967, and was freed March 13. He is now at the Travis Air Force Base medical center.

Mrs. Loretta Stirm's suit asks custody of the couple's four children: Lorrie, 15, Robert Jr., 14, Roger, 12, and Cynthia, 11.

What better photograph and news clipping can depict both the triumph and the tragedy of war!

cream of intelligent leaders of the world were gathered to resolve the conflict. But first, they decided to play a game. Now most people would tire of playing a game after one or two hours.

But these grown men played this game for 8 solid months! The name of the game was:

Shall the table be round
or
Shall the table be square?

At that time Henry Kissinger was the chief negotiator for the U.S.

How can anyone believe that man himself can achieve a Heaven here on earth when it took 8 months of argument just to settle the shape of the peace table in Paris! And the sad aspect of this is that **while they were playing this game...8000 of your sons were killed in Vietnam!**

The Vietnam War, as far as U.S. active participation was concerned, ended on January 27, 1973. Secretary of State William P. Rogers wrote his name 62 times on the documents at last providing a settlement of the longest, most divisive foreign war in America's history—12 years!

And what was the toll?

> Almost 46,000 American dead
> 303,000 American wounded
> $146 billion in military aid

The real toll of the war is just now being felt. The other day, while speaking in a high school auditorium in Plainwell, Michigan...a mother came up to me with tears in her eyes. All she could say is one sentence:

"My son came back from Vietnam with total disability!"

Then, overwhelmed with grief, she ran out the door.

Yesterday's heroes are today's forgotten men. You can find them in government hospitals around the nation...many neglected...lying in dismal wards...bitter...with nothing to live for.

The government cost in post-war benefits will far exceed the cost of the Vietnam War itself.

Yet we were told we had achieved "peace with honor."

Priest Defends Nixon
Aide Calls Profanity Therapeutic

By ROBERT S. BOYD
Inquirer Washington Bureau

WASHINGTON—Stung by charges of immorality in the Oval Office, the White House sent out its resident clergyman Wednesday to defend the morality of President Nixon's confidential conversations on Watergate.

Dr. John McLaughlin, a Jesuit priest and deputy special assistant to the President, said Mr. Nixon's use of profanity and obscenity was "a form of therapy ... with no moral meaning."

Quoting from the Bible and warning against "hypocrisy, sanctimoniousness and selfrighteousness," Father McLaughlin told reporters that the P... being with imperfections, as we all are," but he insisted that, overall, the President has "acquitted himself with honor."

Father McLaughlin's appearance in the office of Ken Clawson, White House director of communications, wearing a gray business suit, was apparently intended to counter mounting criticism of the tone and the content of Mr. Nixon's Watergate conversations as revealed in the book of transcripts published last week.

It was hastily arranged after Senate Republican leader Hugh Scott (Pa.) said in the Senate Tuesday that the transcripts showed "deplorable, disgusting, shabby, immoral per-

---

The Evening Bulletin
SUBURBAN NORTH
INDEPENDENT—LOCALLY OWNED   WITH SUNDAY MORNING EDITION

TUESDAY, MAY 7, 1974   FIFTEEN CENTS

'Shabby, Disgusting, Immoral Performance'
Scott Blasts Nixon Transcripts

By ROBERT E. TAYLOR
Bulletin Washington Bureau

Washington — Sen. Hugh Scott (R-Pa.), the Senate minority leader, today blasted President Nixon's White House transcripts as a "shab... fore the opening of the day's Senate session.

It was his first open criticism of the contents of the transcripts. It marked a major shift in his public stance tow... Scott said of the transcripts today:

"They are a shabby, disgusting, immoral performance. The transcripts have to speak for themselves. I am enormously distressed that there is not enough showing... referring to President Nixon. He said, "I mean by each of those persons (who participated in the conversations) according to what he said."

Despite his expression of moral indignation, Scott said... Nixon on narrow legal grounds.

On Jan. 21, Scott said in a television interview that he "would indicate that on specific items the President would be exculpated entirely."

Graham and the transcripts
'We have lost our moral compass'

By THE REV. BILLY GRAHAM

During the last few days, I set myself to the difficult task of reading the Watergate transcripts, which I have not yet completed. While we have no other President's transcripts by which to compare these, I must confess this has been a profoundly disturbing and disappointing experience. One cannot but deplore the moral tone implied in these papers, and though we know that other Presidents have used equally objectionable language, it does not make it right.

"Thou shalt not take the name of the Lord thy God in vain" is a commandment which has not been suspended, regardless of any need to release tensions. What comes through in these tapes is not the man I have known for many years. After mutual friends have made the same observation.

Now all these matters are in the hands of the judicial process set up by our constitution. The law will take its course.

"What comes through in these tapes is not the man I have known for many years."

—The Rev. Billy Graham

our condemnation of evil must, however, be tempered by compassion for the wrongdoers. Many a stone is being cast by persons whose own lives could not bear like scrutiny. Therefore, we dare not be self-righteous.

A nation confused for years by the teaching of situational ethics now finds itself dismayed by those in government who apparently practiced it. We have lost our moral compass. We must get it

I believe that our nation will survive as a strong and united power. But if we do survive, it will be because we have maintained our moral compass, the law of God. It is by God's moral law that some day we will all be judged.

Therefore, God commands all men everywhere to repent while there is yet time. America needs to repent and turn to God for forgiveness, for correction

In fact, President Nixon, in his ten-minute speech announcing the armistice, called the agreement "peace with honor" five times.

The Real Tragedy Of Watergate

But recent revelations in the Watergate scandal have brought the Presidency to an even lower ebb.

It is my opinion that within the next 30 years events could so occur that the Presidency will be abolished.

On Monday night, May 6, 1974, President Richard Nixon released 1,254 pages and 200,000 words of transcripts of his secret Watergate tapes.

It started on June 17, 1972 when burglars broke into the headquarters of the Democratic Party. At the head of this group was former White House aide, Howard Hunt. Hunt had formerly specialized in secret operations for the CIA.

Of all the revelations which have shocked Americans, none has caused more outrage than that concerning measures authorized by the Presidential staff, violating the privacy and the civil and human rights of citizens.

One thing is clear in the Nixon transcript...the President was willing to consider the use of the Internal Revenue Service, the F.B.I. and the C.I.A. to apply political pressure to achieve his ends. And in certain cases, such pressure was used.

The most distressing part of the Report was not that they show President Nixon guilty necessarily of an impeachable offense. It is in the fact that throughout the entire 200,000 word report it is revealed how totally devoid of moral concern and care for the national welfare of the Nation were the President of the United States and his chief aides!

Nowhere definitively in the Report is there ever a serious question raised as to whether something is ethically right... but rather what is the most politically expedient avenue to take.

Any Bible-believing Christian is further disheartened to discover the constant sprinkling of profanity and obscenity used by the President of the United States. Much of the transcript had to use in parenthesis the words: "(Expletive deleted)."

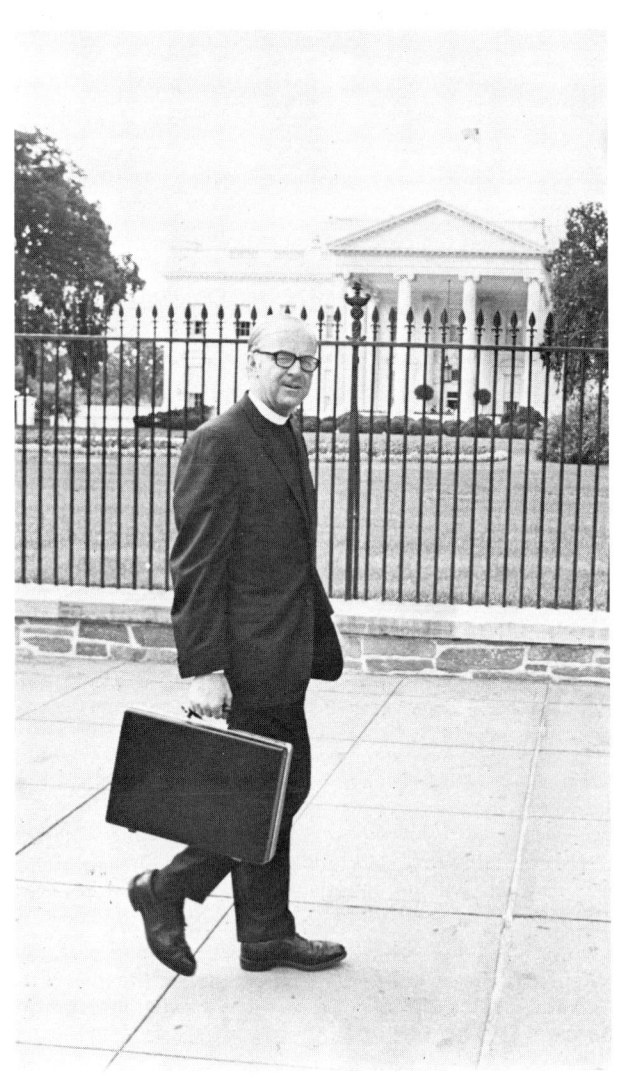

Father John McLaughlin of Providence, Rhode Island, walks along Pennsylvania Avenue past the White House on his way to work in Washington. He is deputy special assistant to the President.

The Strange Alliance

And a further revelation is even more astonishing...and is a prelude of things to come:

Dr. John McLaughlin is a deputy special assistant to the President. He, however, is also a Jesuit priest.

On May 8, 1974 he staunchly defended the President's use of vulgar language...even quoting from the Bible. Among other things McLaughlin said:

> "(the use of such language) was a form of emotional drainage (that is) good, valid and sound.
>
> (Mr. Nixon's use of profanity and obscenity was) a form of therapy...with no moral meaning."

However, Senator Hugh Scott (R. Pa.) referred to the contents of the Nixon Report as a

> "Shabby, disgusting, immoral performance..."

While Rabbi Alexander Schindler, President of the Union of American Hebrew Congregation said the transcripts:

> "...reek with the stench of moral decay...the saddest, most sickening document in the annals of American history."

What is sad is that no important Christian leaders spoke out as forcefully pointing out the sin of these events. There are no modern-day Ezras, no Jeremiahs nor a prophet Nathan to point out sin...even if that path leads right to the doorstep of the Presidency! The age of compromise is here!

And also...the beginning of the end for the United States.

Consider the parallel.

In the hour of Presidential crisis, who represents the President to the people, staunchly defending his use of profanity and obscenity? Who brings it under the cloak of the Bible and surrounding it with verses?

A Clergyman (A Jesuit Priest)

And what is his position?

Deputy Special Assistant to the President!

There may have been a time although I am not aware of

such an instance in recent history, when a President was represented by a clergyman.

But certainly not under such critical conditions and upholding such an anti-Scriptural position!

Prelude To Persecution

Bible-believing Christians should recognize a very inherent danger here. Could this not be the prelude of events leading up to the Tribulation Period?

Are we not seeing a pattern beginning to take shape?

In the Tribulation Period...an impressive leader...the President of the United States of Europe will have a religious counterpart, a religious leader, who will assist him. This religious leader will not try to promote himself but will do all in his power to encourage allegiance to his leader.[1]

There is no doubt in my mind that the Power of the Presidency is rapidly eroding.

In my opinion, it will continue to erode. It will never again have the respect nor the confidence of the people.

In its place we will see an increase in lawlessness, sophisticated crime from kidnappings and bombings to guerrilla warfare, right within the U.S.

I PREDICT that one day before 1980...a homemade nuclear bomb will be exploded in the U.S.

Such uncontrolled crime will bring unprecedented terror in the hearts of the people.

With crime reaching frightening proportions the cry will come for law and order.

And law and order will come...in the form of dictatorial control.

The average age of the world's great civilizations is 200

---

[1] For a complete explanation of the two important powerful personages that take part in the Tribulation Period, we suggest you read GUIDE TO SURVIVAL by Salem Kirban, $2.95. You may order by sending your check to: Salem Kirban, Inc., Kent Road, Huntingdon Valley, Penna. 19006, U.S.A.

years. These nations progressed through this sequence:

> From bondage to spiritual faith
> From spiritual faith to great courage
> From great courage to liberty
> From liberty to abundance
> From abundance to complacency
> From complacency to apathy
> From apathy to dependency
> From dependency back again into bondage.

It was Shakespeare who made Marc Antony say at Caesar's funeral,

If you have tears, prepare to shed them now.

Dedicated or not, the President of the United States will find it impossible to make this country a heaven on earth... nor can he deliver "peace in our time."

Seven years ago I went on a journey in search of peace. Never in my wildest dreams would I have believed that seven years later our country's leaders would so rapidly be heading towards expediency and apathy. It is a brief step from apathy to dependency. And an even briefer one from dependency back again into bondage. And that is our course!

Goodbye Mr. President!

June, 1974
Huntingdon Valley, Pennsylvania

THE JUDGMENTS OF THE TRIBULATION PERIOD

First 3½ Years

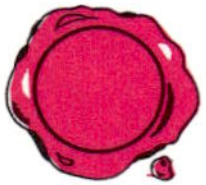

The Seven Seal Judgments
After The Rapture comes....

First Seal	Second Seal	Third Seal	Fourth Seal	Fifth Seal	Sixth Seal	Seventh Seal
Rider on White Horse Peace–Antichrist	Rider on Red Horse War	Rider on Black Horse Famine	Rider on Pale Horse Death	Martyred Souls Persecution	Changes on Earth Destruction	Silence

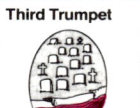

The Seven Trumpet Judgments
From out of the Seventh Seal comes....

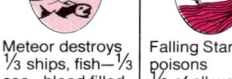

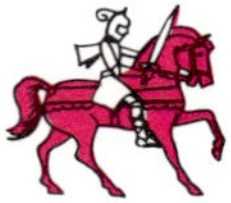

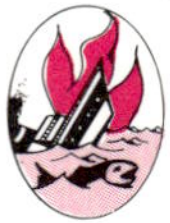

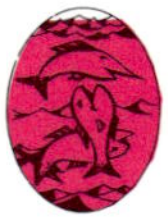

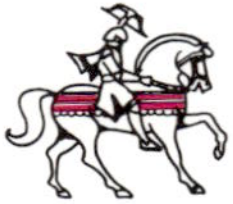

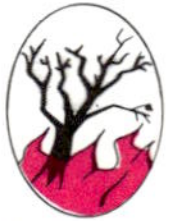

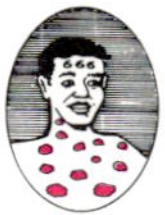

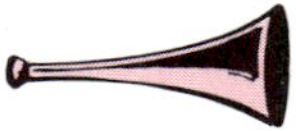

First Trumpet	Second Trumpet	Third Trumpet	Fourth Trumpet	Fifth Trumpet	Sixth Trumpet	Seventh Trumpet
⅓ Earth afire ⅓ Trees burned All grass burned	Meteor destroys ⅓ ships, fish—⅓ sea—blood filled	Falling Star poisons ⅓ of all water	⅓ of sun, moon and stars darkened	5 months of torture by Scorpion stings	Satan's 200 million army kills ⅓ Mankind	Earthquake 7000 die in Jerusalem

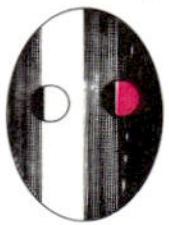

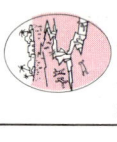

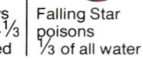

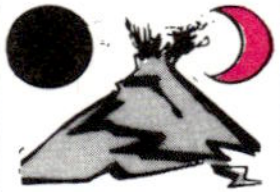

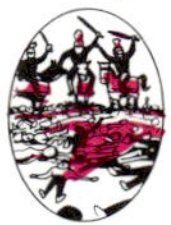

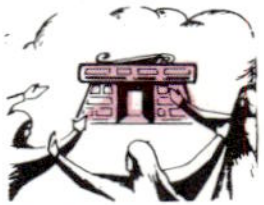

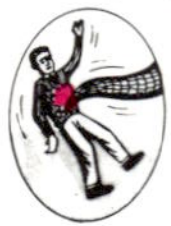

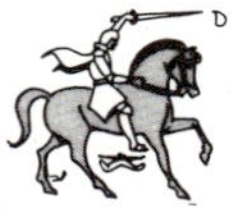

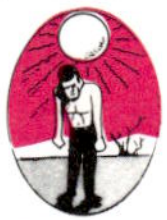

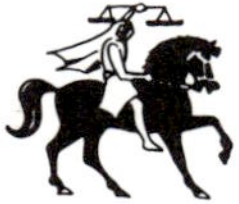

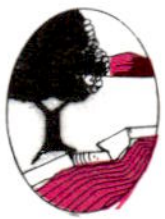

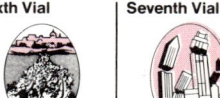

Last 3½ Years

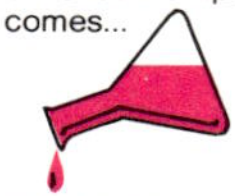

The Seven Vial Judgments
From out of the Seventh Trumpet comes...

First Vial	Second Vial	Third Vial	Fourth Vial	Fifth Vial	Sixth Vial	Seventh Vial
Boils affect those with Mark of Antichrist	Sea of Blood Everything in ocean dies	Rivers of Blood Rivers, springs turn to blood	Heat from Sun scorches all Mankind	Darkness Earth plunged into darkness	River Euphrates Dried up—Army attacks Israel	Hail Cities crumble

Copyright © 1974, Salem Kirban

THE COMING SEQUENCE OF EVENTS
in GOD'S PROPHETIC TIMETABLE

The sequence of events, according to God's Word, the Bible, appears to be as follows:

RAPTURE, including the FIRST RESURRECTION

> This can occur at any time. Believing Christians (both dead and alive) will "in the twinkling of an eye" rise up to meet Christ in the air. Read 1 Thessalonians 4:13-17 and Revelation 20.

TRIBULATION

> This will be a period of 7 years, following the Rapture, of phenomenal world trial and suffering. It is at this time that Antichrist will reign over a federation of 10 nations which quite possibly could include the United States. See Daniel 9:27 and Matthew 24:21.

*BATTLE of ARMAGEDDON

> This will occur at the end of the 7 year Tribulation Period when the Lord Jesus Christ comes down from Heaven and wipes out the combined armies of more than 200 million men. The blood bath covers over 185 miles of Israel. See Revelation 14:20, and 19:11-21.
>
> (While there is a 7 year period of Tribulation on earth ...believers, who have already been raptured into heaven, will stand before their Lord to receive crowns and rewards. Their sins have already been paid for at the cross. See 2 Corinthians 5:10. This is called the **JUDGMENT SEAT OF CHRIST).**

* JUDGMENT of the NATION ISRAEL

> Before the 1000 year Millennium begins all **living** Israel will be regathered in Palestine (Ezekiel 20:35). The unbelievers will be cut off (Ezekiel 20:37) and cast into Hades, and eventually into the Lake of Fire (Matthew 25:30). The believers, those who have accepted Jesus Christ as Messiah and Lord, will be taken into the Millennium (Ezekiel 20:40-44).

*JUDGMENT of the GENTILES

> Before the 1000 year Millennium but after the Judgment of the Nation Israel...all **living** Gentiles who have survived the Tribulation Period will be regathered in Jerusalem (Joel 3:2; Zechariah 14:4). The unbelievers will be cast into Hades, and eventually into the Lake of Fire (Matthew 25:41). The believers, those who have accepted Jesus Christ as Saviour and

Lord, will live on earth for the Millennium Period (Matthew 25:34).

*RESURRECTION of the TRIBULATION SAINTS

Those who have accepted Christ during the Tribulation Period will be raised from the dead by the close of the Tribulation's 7 years as part of the First Resurrection (Daniel 12:1-2 and Revelation 20).

*DISPOSITION OF EVIL ONES

During this same period...at the end of the Tribulation...Antichrist and the False Prophet are thrown into the Lake of Fire (Revelation 19:20).

Satan is bound in the bottomless pit for 1000 years (Revelation 20:1-3).

*MILLENNIUM (1000 Years) REIGN OF CHRIST

This is a period when all the believers of all the ages reign with Christ. Those previously resurrected in the Rapture and those saints who died in the Tribulation and were *resurrected*...will reign with Christ in the Millennial Age as **Resurrected believers.** They will be given positions of responsibility in the Millennial Kingdom (Matthew 19:28, Luke 19:12-27).

The saved of Israel will again be in a position of prominence (Isaiah 49:22-23). They will be given positions of leadership (Isaiah 61:5-6). Gentiles and Jews alike who are still *living* at the close of the Battle of Armageddon, and who are permitted to enter the Millennial Kingdom, are known as **Living Believers.** These were not raptured (they were not believers at the time of the Rapture), nor did they die in the Tribulation period (they survived). They are still in their human unresurrected bodies.

During the Millennium these **Living Believers** will still be able to reproduce children. Children born of these Living Believers will still be born with a sin nature. And for them, salvation is still required. They must individually make a decision whether to accept Jesus Christ as Saviour and Lord...or to deny Him (Ezekiel 36:37-38; Jeremiah 30:19-20).

* THE FINAL REBELLION

At the end of the 1000 year Millennium Period, Satan will have a brief and last opportunity to deceive people. You must remember that many will be born during the Millennial Period. Millions will follow Satan. This vast number of people will completely encircle the Living Believers within Jerusalem in a state of siege.

When this occurs, God brings fire down from Heaven killing the millions of Satan's army (Revelation 20).

* GREAT WHITE THRONE JUDGMENT

This is when the unsaved, non-believers, of all of the ages are resurrected and are judged before God. These are condemned forever to the Lake of Fire. Both living (from the Millennium) and dead **unsaved** are judged here. Those previously dead, up to this point, have already been in hell in torment, awaiting this Final Judgment Day (Revelation 20:11-15).

EARTH BURNS UP

To purify this earth, so tainted with the scars of sin, God sets it afire with a fervent heat. See 2 Peter 3:7,10.

The NEW HEAVENS and the NEW EARTH

All Christians finally reach the ultimate in glory reigning forever with Christ in a new heaven and a new earth (Revelation 21).

The novel **666** by Salem Kirban covers the Tribulation Period. Those time periods preceded by an asterisk (*) are the area that the novel **1000** covers. Chapter 1 of the book **1000** by Salem Kirban begins with the final stages of the Battle of Armageddon. **GUIDE TO SURVIVAL** covers current events leading up to the Rapture and also details the Tribulation Period. **YOUR LAST GOODBYE** includes current events that are drawing us close to the end times as well as covers the 1000-year Millennium and the New Heavens and New Earth.

WHAT WILL YOU DO WITH JESUS?

After reading this book it should become evident to you that the world is **not** getting better and better.

What happens when it comes time for you to depart from this earth?

Then WHAT WILL YOU DO WITH JESUS?

Here are five basic observations in the Bible of which you should be aware:

1. ALL SIN — For all have sinned, and come short of the glory of God. (Romans 3:23)
2. ALL LOVED — For God so loved the world, that He gave His only begotten Son, that whosoever believeth in Him should not perish, but have everlasting life (John 3:16)
3. ALL RAISED — Marvel not at this: for the hour is coming, in which all that are in the graves shall hear his voice,

    And shall come forth; they that have done good, unto the resurrection of life; and they that have done evil, unto the resurrection of damnation. (John 5:28,29)
4. ALL JUDGED — ...we shall all stand before the judgment seat of Christ. (Romans 14:10)

    And I saw the dead, small and great, stand before God; and the books were opened...(Revelation 20:12)
5. ALL BOW — ...at the name of Jesus every knee should bow...(Philippians 2:10)

Right now, in simple faith, you can have the wonderful assurance of eternal life.

Ask yourself, honestly, the question....WHAT WILL I DO WITH JESUS?

God tells us the following:

"...him that cometh to me I will in no wise cast out. (37) Verily, verily (truly) I say unto you, He that believeth on me (Christ) *hath* everlasting life" (47)—(John 6:37, 47).

He also is a righteous God and a God of indignation to those who reject Him....

"...he that believeth not is condemned already, because he hath not believed in the name of the only begotten Son of God"—(John 3:18).

"And whosoever was not found written in the book of life was cast into the lake of fire"—(Revelation 20:15).

YOUR MOST IMPORTANT DECISION IN LIFE

All of your riches here on earth—all of your financial security—all of your material wealth, your houses, your land will crumble into nothingness in a few years.

No matter how great your works—no matter how kind you are—no matter how philanthropic you are—it means nothing in the sight of God, because in the sight of God, your riches are as filthy rags.

"...all our righteousnesses are as filthy rags..." (Isaiah 64:6)

Christ expects you to come as you are, a sinner, recognizing your need of a Saviour, the Lord Jesus Christ.

Understanding this, why not bow your head right now and give this simple prayer of faith to the Lord.

My Personal Decision for CHRIST

"Lord Jesus, I know that I'm a sinner and that I cannot save myself by good works. I believe that you died for me and that you shed your blood for my sins. I believe that you rose again from the dead. And now I am receiving you as my personal Saviour, my Lord, my only hope of salvation. I know that I cannot save myself. Lord, be merciful to me, a sinner, and save me according to the promise of Your Word. I want Christ to come into my heart now to be my Saviour, Lord and Master."

Signed ....

Date ....

If you have signed the above, having just taken Christ as your personal Saviour and Lord...I would like to rejoice with you in your new found faith.

Write to me...Salem Kirban, Kent Road, Huntingdon Valley, Penna. 19006...and I'll send you a little booklet to help you start living your new life in Christ.

LIFE BEGAN FOR ME AT 42

I will never forget that day I stood in a mortuary in Vietnam and witnessed some 50 servicemen—dead, getting ready to be processed for their last journey home!

Tears came to my eyes as I said to myself:

> Lord...what's wrong with me?
> It's too late to tell these young men...18, 19, 20 years of age...that Jesus died so they might have life.
> If they haven't already accepted Christ as Saviour and Lord, they are destined for an eternity in Hell!

> Lord, I accepted Jesus Christ as my personal Saviour at 8 years of age at Montrose Bible Conference in Montrose, Pennsylvania.

> I heard such great speakers as Alexander Graham Scroggie, Harry Ironsides and Will Houghton...who was then President of Moody Bible Institute.

> Will Houghton, who wrote that famous chorus:

>> Lead me to some soul today,
>> Oh teach me Lord just what to say
>> Friends of mine are lost in sin
>> And cannot find their way!

My thoughts continued:

Lord, from 8 years of age until now I have been playing at Christianity. Oh yes, I have been active in my church; President of the Young People's fellowship, President of our Choir, gave liberally to my Church. If I had died, they would have said, "He was a tremendous Christian!"

But I wasn't. I was playing Church...more concerned about material gains than the souls of men!

Some 9000 miles from home, the Lord convicted me of my complacency!

And life began for me at 42 years of age in a mortuary in Vietnam!

Right now as **you** read these words, I don't care how old you are — 15, 17, 18, 21, 25, 33, 42, 48, 54, 59, 62, 68, or 75...

Life can begin triumphantly **this very moment** for you...or you can continue to live the same dull routine life of going to church on Sunday and then living for self and material gain the rest of the week.

The story is told about East Berlin and West Berlin.

East Berlin is communist controlled. West Berlin is free.

The people in East Berlin
   got a truckload of garbage...
   and dumped it on the West Berlin side!

The people in West Berlin could have done the same thing.

Instead, they got a truckload of
   butter and eggs, canned goods and honey
   and neatly stacked it on the East Berlin side
   with this sign.

EACH GIVES WHAT HE HAS!

Honestly now...why not this very moment, get down on your hands and knees and pray to God.

Search your heart. What has your life been like since you accepted Jesus Christ as Saviour and Lord of your life?

Have you been giving him the garbage of your life?

If you have, wouldn't you now like to start giving him the butter, the eggs, the canned goods and honey?

EACH

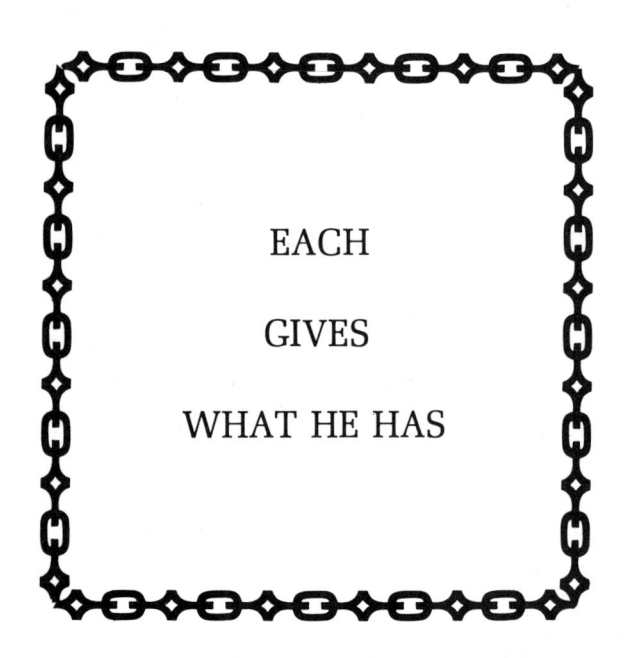

GIVES

WHAT HE HAS

Top photo:
Salem Kirban with wife,
Mary, June 1972

Bottom photo:
Author's wedding day,
August 17, 1946

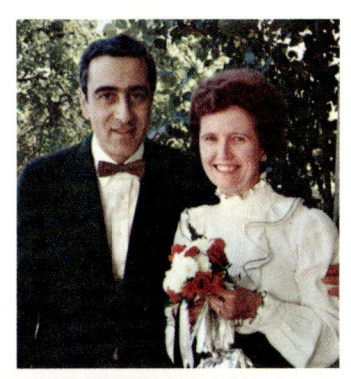

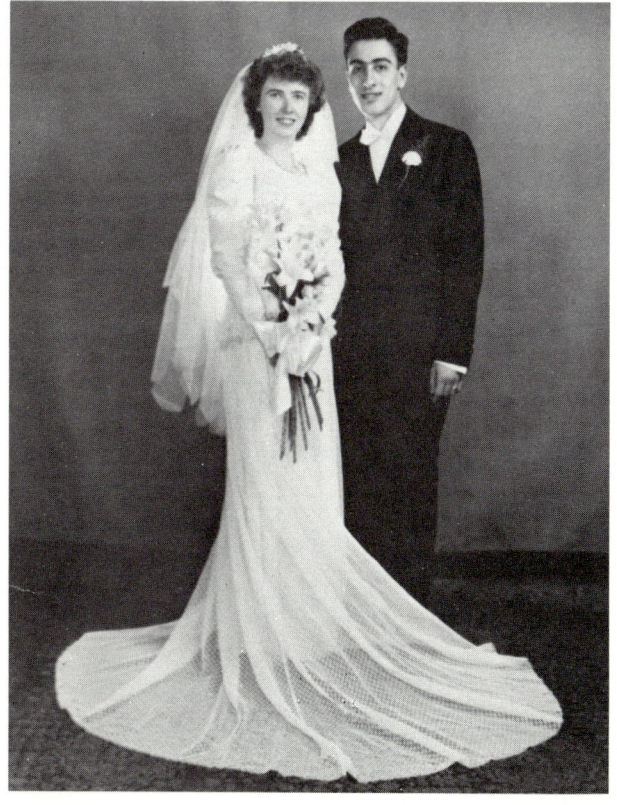

Have you ever told **anyone** you are personally interested in their soul? Are you so concerned about something good happening **to you** that you have failed to tell those without Christ...that something good...eternal life...could happen **to them!**

LIFE BEGAN FOR ME at 42! Up until that time I had not written one book! Since then...some 7 years...I have written some 22 books. Each book has as its last chapter a Decision Chapter pointing the reader to Christ. That is the sole purpose of my writing...to win souls from an eternity in Hell to an ever glorious eternity in God's Heaven!

What is your sole purpose in life?

If you are tired of giving Christ the garbage of your life and you now want to give him your best...it may mean you will have to change your whole pattern of living and giving.

But you will find no greater joy...
   than the joy of serving Jesus!

You will find no greater thrill...
   than the thrill of seeing lives
   redeemed from sin to life everlasting
And all because YOU CARE!

Won't you pray this prayer with me found on the following page, right now?

If you have signed **MY DAY OF DEDICATION...**
I would like to rejoice with you in your moment of decision.

Write to me...Salem Kirban, Kent Road, Huntingdon Valley, Pennsylvania 19006, U.S.A. Your letter will have made this book singularly worthwhile!

MY DAY OF DEDICATION

Precious Lord Jesus,
I realize I have been more concerned
 about myself and less about others.

I have been playing at Christianity,
 satisfied to give you the garbage of
 my life...while I held on to the
 butter, eggs, canned goods and honey.

Now, this very moment, I want
 life with meaning,
 joy through serving,
 fulfillment through fulfilling.

Material ambitions and selfish desires
 I now place behind me.

Give me courage to tell others the precious
 joy of eternal life that you have shared
 with me. Give me a burden for my loved
 ones, my neighbors, my world.

For in telling,
 Give me a harvest.

And in harvest,
 Give me matchless joy.

And in joy,
 eternal peace and contentment

For in giving...there is receiving
And in receiving...there is Crowning!

Forgive me Lord for my sin of indifference.
Use me Lord as your channel of love.

Today...at age _____

This day _____
        Day   Month   Year

I want to start really living **now** for the Lord.

I WANT LIFE TO BEGIN FOR ME...Triumphantly!

_____
Sign your name

DATE DUE

ORTHOGRAPHE RECOMMANDÉE

EXERCICES
et mots courants

**Orthographe recommandée :
exercices et mots courants**
par Chantal Contant

ISBN 978-2-9808720-5-1

Le contenu de ce livre est applicable dans toute la francophonie.

Conception et rédaction : Chantal Contant
Couverture : Christian Dugas

Dépôt légal :
Bibliothèque et Archives nationales du Québec, 2011
Bibliothèque et Archives Canada, 2011
Bibliothèque nationale de France, 2011

Tous droits réservés
© Chantal Contant 2011
www.chantalcontant.info

www.**orthographe-recommandee**.info

Éditeur :
De Champlain S. F.
6455, rue Jean-Talon Est, bureau 1002
Montréal (Québec) H1S 3E8 — Canada
livres@dechamplain.ca

Imprimé au Canada par Marquis imprimeur inc.

Autres ouvrages sur l'orthographe : voir les pages 193 à 200 et la bibliographie à la page 212.

Chantal Contant

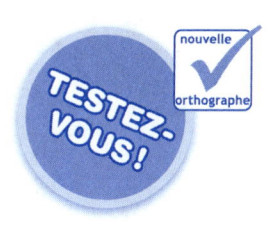

TESTEZ-VOUS !

nouvelle orthographe ✓

ORTHOGRAPHE RECOMMANDÉE

EXERCICES
et mots courants

De Champlain S. F.

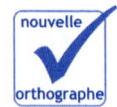

© Chantal Contant 2011

Conformément aux lois relatives aux droits d'auteur, toute reproduction, par quelque procédé que ce soit, et sans accord préalable écrit de l'éditeur, est strictement interdite.

Défiez l'orthographe !

Doit-on écrire :
- ☐ **shampoing** ou ☐ **shampooing** ?
- ☐ **froufrou** ou ☐ **frou-frou** ?
- ☐ **acuponcture** ou ☐ **acupuncture** ?
- ☐ **des allume-feux** ou ☐ **des allume-feu** ?

Toutes ces formes existent en français, mais celles de gauche sont recommandées.

Avec ce livre, vous découvrirez :
- ☑ la **forme recommandée** d'un mot ;
- ☑ la **règle** d'orthographe.

70 tests, exercices, jeux

Amusez-vous à choisir entre les formes **a** ou **b**, à démêler le vrai du faux, à faire des jeux...

500 mots courants

Parcourez la liste de 500 mots fréquents afin de bien visualiser l'orthographe recommandée.

Les difficultés orthographiques

L'orthographe française est capricieuse, mais elle respecte aussi des règles.

Certaines de ces règles sont plus récentes et elles ont été mises en place pour corriger des exceptions inutiles.

Il y a vingt ou trente ans, pourquoi écrivait-on :
- **trémolo** mais **mod_e_rato** ?
- **imbécile** mais **imbéci_ll_ité** ?
- **souffler** mais **boursou_f_ler** ?
- **combattre** mais **comba_t_if** ?
- **un millefeuille** mais **un mill_e_-pattes** ?
- **extracorporel** mais **extr_a_-courant** ?

Ces incohérences ne faisaient que surcharger la mémoire et défiaient toute logique. Elles sont maintenant rectifiées* grâce à de nouvelles règles officielles.

---

*Aujourd'hui, des dictionnaires comme le *Larousse des noms communs*, le *Petit Robert*, le *Dictionnaire Hachette* et le *Nouveau Littré* reconnaissent les formes plus régulières **modérato**, **imbécilité**, **boursouffler**, **combattif**, **un millepatte** et **extracourant**. Les correcteurs de Word, d'OpenOffice.org et d'Antidote les ont intégrées aussi. Ces nouvelles formes sont donc admises. À nous tous de les utiliser maintenant.

Une orthographe recommandée

Le **Conseil supérieur** de la langue française à Paris a mis en place ces nouvelles règles officielles. L'**Académie** française les approuve.

Les **dictionnaires** et **correcteurs** se mettent à jour (détails au www.nouvelleorthographe.info).

Les ministères de l'**Éducation** des principaux pays de la francophonie les reconnaissent : **France**, **Belgique**, **Québec**, **Suisse** (voir le www.orthographe-recommandee.info/enseignement).

À vos marques, partez !

À votre tour de découvrir ces règles.

Commencez par le test intuitif : il sert à voir si, spontanément, vous écrivez déjà en appliquant la nouvelle orthographe. Ce test ne vous demande pas quelle est « la » bonne réponse, mais comment vous écrivez. Et attention : certains choix de réponses sont fautifs...

Certains exercices sembleront faciles. C'est normal, et tant mieux ! Vous voulez maitriser* les plus récentes règles orthographiques, pas vous faire piéger avec d'anciennes exceptions.

---

*On écrit maintenant **maitriser** sans accent circonflexe.

TESTEZ-VOUS!

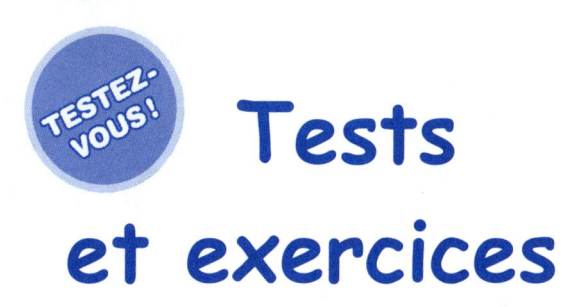

Tests et exercices

Chaque règle sera explorée par étapes :

- Étape 1 ☑☐☐☐
  Je me teste (test intuitif)

- Étape 2 ☑☑☐☐
  Je découvre (règle)

- Étape 3 ☑☑☑☐
  Je m'exerce (exercices de compréhension)

- Étape 4 ☑☑☑☑
  Je corrige (réponses)

Les règles ont été regroupées en six thèmes, suivis chaque fois d'une série d'activités de type « *VRAI* ou *FAUX* », d'exercices récapitulatifs ou de jeux.

Bonne exploration !

Le trait d'union et la soudure

RÈGLES **A**

trait d'union et soudure | singulier et pluriel | accents et tréma

par Chantal Contant

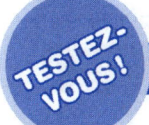

TESTEZ-VOUS!

Étape 1 ☑☐☐☐   RÈGLE A1

Je me teste

TEST INTUITIF

Encerclez la forme que <u>vous</u> employez.

▶ En rédigeant, j'écrirais spontanément…

1. a) du contre-plaqué   b) du contreplaqué
2. a) un contre-poison   b) un contrepoison
3. a) un contre-exemple   b) un contrexemple
4. a) une contre-attaque   b) une contrattaque
5. a) un contre-la-montre   b) un contrelamontre
6. a) s'entre-détruire   b) s'entredétruire
7. a) s'entre-tuer   b) s'entretuer
8. a) entr'apercevoir   b) entrapercevoir
9. a) de l'entr'aide   b) de l'entraide
10. a) l'entre-jambes   b) l'entrejambe

Voyez le corrigé (p. 201-202) et comparez vos réponses. Vous employez probablement **déjà** certaines graphies recommandées.

Découvrez maintenant à l'étape 2 la règle de la soudure avec **contr**(**e**)- et **entr**(**e**)-.

---

consonnes doubles   anomalies rectifiées   choix recommandés

Étape 2 ☑☑☐☐ RÈGLE A1

Je découvre

NON RECOMMANDÉ	RECOMMANDÉ
contre-culture	**contreculture**
contre-indication	**contrindication**
un entre-deux	**un entredeux**
s'entr'aimer	**s'entraimer**

J'apprends — Soudure

On écrit sans trait d'union les mots composés avec les préfixes **contr(e)-** et **entr(e)-**.

J'ai déjà vu ça — La règle existait en partie

On avait déjà **contredire**, **contrepoids**, **entrecouper**, **entremêler** en un seul mot.

J'observe — Le e s'efface

Le **e** disparait devant voyelle : **contrappel**, **contrindiqué**, **s'entrégorger**, **entrouvrir**.

Je note — Ne pas souder trois mots

Cette règle ne touche pas des mots comme **contre-la-montre** et **entre-deux-guerres** (pas de préfixe dans ces cas composés de trois mots).

trait d'union et soudure | singulier et pluriel | accents et tréma

par Chantal Contant

Étape 3 ☑☑☑☐ **RÈGLE A1**

Je m'exerce

SOUDURE AVEC **CONTR(E)-** ET **ENTR(E)-**

Niveau de difficulté : ★☆☆☆☆

Encerclez la forme recommandée.

▶ Selon la règle, il est préférable d'écrire…

11. a) **en contre-plongée** b) **en contreplongée**
12. a) **contre-espionnage** b) **contrespionnage**
13. a) **s'entre-déchirer** b) **s'entredéchirer**
14. a) **entr'ouvrir** b) **entrouvrir**
15. a) **s'entre-haïr** b) **s'entrehaïr**
16. a) **l'entre-deux-guerres** b) **l'entredeuxguerres**
17. a) **à contre-jour** b) **à contrejour**
18. a) **contre-offensive** b) **controffensive**
19. a) **entre-temps** b) **entretemps**
20. a) **contre-interroger** b) **contrinterroger**

Les réponses sont données à l'étape 4 (p. 14).

Ma note : /10

---

consonnes doubles anomalies rectifiées choix recommandés

Étape 4 ☑☑☑ **RÈGLE A1**

Je corrige

SOUDURE AVEC **CONTR(E)-** ET **ENTR(E)-**

Voici le corrigé des pages 11 et 13.

La réponse est **b)** pour tous les numéros sauf 5 et 16 : **du contreplaqué**, **un contrepoison**, **un contrexemple**, **une contrattaque**, **s'entredétruire**, **s'entretuer**, **entrapercevoir**, **de l'entraide**, **l'entrejambe**, **en contreplongée**, **contrespionnage**, **s'entredéchirer**, **entrouvrir**, **s'entrehaïr**, **à contrejour**, **controffensive**, **entretemps**, **contrinterroger**.

La réponse est **a)** aux numéros **5** et **16** : **un contre-la-montre**, **l'entre-deux-guerres**.

⊗ La forme donnée en **2a** n'existe pas, car **contrepoison** s'écrit toujours en un seul mot. La forme donnée en **9a** n'existe plus de nos jours, car les dictionnaires modernes écrivent **entraide** en un mot. Par contre, les graphies soudées **5b** (dans le test) et **16b** (dans l'exercice) sont interdites. Rayez ces quatre formes inexistantes : 2a, 5b, 9a, 16b.

✓ Fin de la règle A1.

| trait d'union et soudure | singulier et pluriel | accents et tréma |

TESTEZ-VOUS!

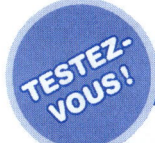

Étape 1 ☑☐☐☐   RÈGLE A2

Je me teste

TEST INTUITIF

Encerclez la forme que <u>vous</u> employez.

▶ En rédigeant, j'écrirais spontanément...

1. a) **extra-terrestre**   b) **extraterrestre**
2. a) **extra-fort**   b) **extrafort**
3. a) **extra-institutionnel**   b) **extrainstitutionnel**
4. a) **extra-ordinaire**   b) **extraordinaire**
5. a) **infra-rouge**   b) **infrarouge**
6. a) **intra-artériel**   b) **intraartériel**
7. a) **intra-utérin**   b) **intrautérin**
8. a) **intra-veineuse**   b) **intraveineuse**
9. a) **ultra-chic**   b) **ultrachic**
10. a) **ultra-violet**   b) **ultraviolet**

Voyez le corrigé (p. 201-202) et comparez vos réponses. Vous employez probablement **déjà** certaines graphies recommandées.

Découvrez maintenant à l'étape 2 la règle avec **extra-**, **infra-**, **intra-** et **ultra-**.

consonnes doubles   anomalies rectifiées   choix recommandés

Étape 2 ☑☑☐☐ — RÈGLE A2

Je découvre

NON RECOMMANDÉ	RECOMMANDÉ
extra-fin	**extrafin**
infra-acoustique	**infraacoustique**
intra-veineux	**intraveineux**
ultra-secret	**ultrasecret**

J'apprends — Soudure

On écrit en un mot les mots composés avec les préfixes **extra-**, **infra-**, **intra-** et **ultra-**.

J'ai déjà vu ça — La règle existait en partie

En effet, on rencontrait déjà **extrajudiciaire**, **extraordinaire**, **infrarouge**, **intracellulaire**, **ultraléger**, **ultrason** en un mot dans les dictionnaires.

Je note — Ne pas souder a+i ni a+u

Le trait d'union est maintenu dans les mots où la soudure engendrerait un problème de prononciation, c'est-à-dire si **a** est suivi de **i** ou de **u**, pour éviter les sons **ai**, **ain** et **au**. Exemples : **intra-image**, **intra-individuel**, **intra-universitaire**, **extra-utérin**.

trait d'union et soudure | singulier et pluriel | accents et tréma

par Chantal Contant

Étape 3 ☑☑☑☐ **RÈGLE A2**

Je m'exerce

SOUDURE AVEC **EXTRA-**, **INFRA-**, **INTRA-** ET **ULTRA-**

Niveau de difficulté : ★★☆☆☆

Encerclez la forme recommandée.

▶ Selon la règle, il est préférable d'écrire...

11. a) **ultra-sensible** b) **ultrasensible**
12. a) **intra-individuel** b) **intraindividuel**
13. a) **intra-atomique** b) **intraatomique**
14. a) **infra-son** b) **infrason**
15. a) **extra-atmosphérique** b) **extraatmosphérique**
16. a) **extra-parlementaire** b) **extraparlementaire**
17. a) **extra-lucide** b) **extralucide**
18. a) **ultra-révolutionnaire** b) **ultrarévolutionnaire**
19. a) **ultra-mince** b) **ultramince**
20. a) **intra-oculaire** b) **intraoculaire**

Les réponses sont données à l'étape 4 (p. 18).

Ma note :   /10

consonnes doubles   anomalies rectifiées   choix recommandés

Étape 4 ☑☑☑   RÈGLE A2

Je corrige

SOUDURE AVEC **EXTRA-**, **INFRA-**, **INTRA-** ET **ULTRA-**

Voici le corrigé des pages 15 et 17.

La réponse est **b)** pour tous les numéros sauf 3, 7 et 12 : **extraterrestre**, **extrafort**, **extraordinaire**, **infrarouge**, **intraartériel**, **intraveineuse**, **ultrachic**, **ultraviolet**, **ultrasensible**, **intraatomique**, **infrason**, **extraatmosphérique**, **extraparlementaire**, **extralucide**, **ultrarévolutionnaire**, **ultramince**, **intraoculaire**.

La réponse est **a)** aux numéros **3**, **7** et **12** : **extra-institutionnel**, **intra-utérin**, **intra-individuel**.

⊗ Les formes données en **a)** aux numéros 5, 8 à 11, 14 et 16 à 20 n'existent plus : de nos jours, les dictionnaires écrivent en un mot **infrarouge**, **intraveineuse**, **ultrachic**, **ultraviolet**, **ultrasensible**, **infrason**, **extraparlementaire**, **extralucide**, **ultrarévolutionnaire**, **ultramince**, **intraoculaire**. Et **4a** n'existe pas, car **extraordinaire** s'écrit toujours en un mot. Les soudures **3b**, **7b** et **12b** sont interdites. Rayez-les.

✓ Fin de la règle A2.

trait d'union et soudure   singulier et pluriel   accents et tréma

par Chantal Contant

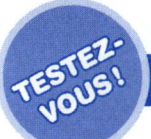

TESTEZ-VOUS !

Étape 1 ☑☐☐☐   **RÈGLE A3**

Je me teste

TEST INTUITIF

Encerclez la forme que <u>vous</u> employez.

▶ En rédigeant, j'écrirais spontanément…

1. a) **cardio-vasculaire**   b) **cardiovasculaire**
2. a) **socio-économique**   b) **socioéconomique**
3. a) **neuro-imagerie**   b) **neuroimagerie**
4. a) **mini-jupe**   b) **minijupe**
5. a) **anti-pollution**   b) **antipollution**
6. a) **franco-britannique**   b) **francobritannique**
7. a) **bio-dégradable**   b) **biodégradable**
8. a) **hydro-électrique**   b) **hydroélectrique**
9. a) **micro-ondes**   b) **microonde**
10. a) **co-fondateur**   b) **cofondateur**

Voyez le corrigé (p. 201-202) et comparez vos réponses. Vous employez probablement **déjà** certaines graphies recommandées.

Découvrez maintenant à l'étape 2 la règle de la soudure avec des éléments savants.

---

consonnes doubles   anomalies rectifiées   choix recommandés

Étape 2 ☑☑☐☐ — RÈGLE A3

Je découvre

NON RECOMMANDÉ	RECOMMANDÉ
anti-brouillard	**antibrouillard**
médico-légal	**médicolégal**
mini-golf	**minigolf**
socio-culturel	**socioculturel**

J'apprends — Soudure

On écrit sans trait d'union les mots composés d'éléments savants (en particulier en **o**) comme **électro-**, **hydro-**, **socio-**, **anti-**…

Je note — Ne pas souder a+i, a+u, o+i, o+u

On maintient le trait d'union pour éviter une prononciation fautive si **a** ou **o** est suivi de **i** ou de **u** (on évite **ai**, **ain**, **au**, **oi**, **oin** et **ou**). Ex. : **micro-informatique**, **mono-usager**.

Je fais attention — Noms géographiques

On maintient le trait d'union lorsqu'il sert à marquer une relation de coordination entre des termes désignant des noms propres ou géographiques. Exemples : **italo-russe**, **anglo-saxon**, **franco-belge**, **serbo-croate**.

---

trait d'union et soudure | singulier et pluriel | accents et tréma

Étape 3 ☑☑☑☐ — RÈGLE A3

Je m'exercice

SOUDURE AVEC DES ÉLÉMENTS SAVANTS

Niveau de difficulté : ★★☆☆☆

Encerclez la forme recommandée.

▶ Selon la règle, il est préférable d'écrire...

11. a) **audio-visuel** b) **audiovisuel**
12. a) **auto-apprentissage** b) **autoapprentissage**
13. a) **gréco-romain** b) **grécoromain**
14. a) **bio-industrie** b) **bioindustrie**
15. a) **maniaco-dépressif** b) **maniacodépressif**
16. a) **cumulo-nimbus** b) **cumulonimbus**
17. a) **ciné-parc** b) **cinéparc**
18. a) **néo-classique** b) **néoclassique**
19. a) **post-référendaire** b) **postréférendaire**
20. a) **télé-objectif** b) **téléobjectif**

Les réponses sont données à l'étape 4 (p. 22).

Ma note :   /10

consonnes doubles   anomalies rectifiées   choix recommandés

Étape 4 ☑☑☑☑ — RÈGLE A3

Je corrige

Soudure avec des éléments savants

Voici le corrigé des pages 19 et 21.

La réponse est **b)** pour tous les numéros sauf 3, 6, 13 et 14 : **cardiovasculaire, socioéconomique, minijupe, antipollution, biodégradable, hydroélectrique, microonde, cofondateur, audiovisuel, autoapprentissage, maniacodépressif, cumulonimbus, cinéparc, néoclassique, postréférendaire, téléobjectif**.

La réponse est **a)** aux numéros **3**, **6**, **13** et **14** : **neuro-imagerie** (évite **oi**), **franco-britannique**, **gréco-romain** (relations de coordination), **bio-industrie** (évite **oin**).

⊗ Les formes données en **7a**, **10a**, **12a** et **16a** n'existent plus : de nos jours, les dictionnaires écrivent en un seul mot les termes composés de **bio-**, de **co-**, de **auto-** et de **cumulo-** (sauf devant **i** et **u**). Les graphies soudées **3b**, **6b**, **13b** et **14b** sont interdites. Rayez-les dans le test et dans l'exercice.

✓ Fin de la règle A3.

trait d'union et soudure | singulier et pluriel | accents et tréma

par Chantal Contant

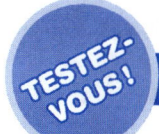

TESTEZ-VOUS!

Étape 1 ☑☐☐☐   RÈGLE A4

Je me teste

TEST INTUITIF

Encerclez la forme que <u>vous</u> employez.

▶ En rédigeant, j'écrirais spontanément…

1. a) **tam-tam**   b) **tamtam**
2. a) **frou-frou**   b) **froufrou**
3. a) **coin-coin**   b) **coincoin**
4. a) **guili-guili**   b) **guiliguili**
5. a) **base-ball**   b) **baseball**
6. a) **hot dog**   b) **hotdog**
7. a) **statu quo**   b) **statuquo**
8. a) **bossa-nova**   b) **bossanova**
9. a) **prima donna**   b) **primadonna**
10. a) **osso-buco**   b) **ossobuco**

Voyez les réponses à la page 202. Combien de formes modernes avez-vous choisies sur 10 ?

Découvrez à l'étape 2 la règle de la soudure des onomatopées et des mots empruntés à d'autres langues.

---

consonnes doubles   anomalies rectifiées   choix recommandés

24 Orthographe recommandée : exercices et mots courants

Étape 2 ☑☑☐☐   RÈGLE A4

Je découvre

NON RECOMMANDÉ	RECOMMANDÉ
bla-bla ou **bla bla**	**blabla**
tic-tac ou **tic tac**	**tictac**
basket-ball	**basketball**
hara-kiri	**harakiri**

J'apprends   Soudure

On écrit en un seul mot les onomatopées* et des mots d'origine étrangère bien implantés dans l'usage.

*Une onomatopée est un mot imitatif, souvent répétitif, évoquant un bruit (ex. : **cuicui**).

J'ai déjà vu ça   La règle existait en partie

On trouvait déjà des mots comme **glouglou** ou **football** écrits sans trait d'union.

J'observe   Le pluriel se régularise

Ces mots étant devenus des mots simples, ils suivent la règle générale du pluriel. Par exemple : **des tictacs**, **des primadonnas**.

trait d'union et soudure | singulier et pluriel | accents et tréma

par Chantal Contant

Étape 3 ☑☑☑☐ **RÈGLE A4**

Je m'exerce

SOUDURE : ONOMATOPÉES ET MOTS EMPRUNTÉS

Niveau de difficulté : ★☆☆☆☆

Encerclez la forme recommandée.

▶ Selon la règle, il est préférable d'écrire...

11. a) **tchin-tchin** b) **tchintchin**
12. a) **hi-han** b) **hihan**
13. a) **cui-cui** b) **cuicui**
14. a) **cha-cha-cha** b) **chachacha**
15. a) **water-polo** b) **waterpolo**
16. a) **un don Juan** b) **un donjuan**
17. a) **fox-trot** b) **foxtrot**
18. a) **spina-bifida** b) **spinabifida**
19. a) **week-end** b) **weekend**
20. a) **volley-ball** b) **volleyball**

Les réponses sont données à l'étape 4.

Ma note :   /10

consonnes doubles   anomalies rectifiées   choix recommandés

Étape 4 ☑☑☑ **RÈGLE A4**

Je corrige

SOUDURE : ONOMATOPÉES ET MOTS EMPRUNTÉS

Voici le corrigé des pages 23 et 25.

La réponse est **b)** pour tous les numéros : **tamtam, froufrou, coincoin, guiliguili, baseball, hotdog, statuquo, bossanova, primadonna, ossobuco, tchintchin, hihan, cuicui, chachacha, waterpolo, un donjuan, foxtrot, spinabifida, weekend, volleyball**.

Note : La règle A4 inclut aussi des termes comme ceux de la liste ci-dessous :

bipbip	**gnangnan**	**teufteuf**
bouiboui	**gouzigouzi**	**toctoc**
cachecache	**grigri**	**tohubohu**
cahincaha	**kifkif**	**traintrain**
cotcot	**mélimélo**	**tralala**
coucicouça	**neuneu**	**troutrou**
cricri	**pêlemêle**	**tsétsé**
daredare	**prêchiprêcha**	**tsointsoin**
flafla	**ricrac**	**yéyé**

✓ Fin de la règle A4.

trait d'union et soudure | singulier et pluriel | accents et tréma

par Chantal Contant

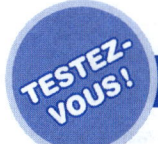

TESTEZ-VOUS !

Étape 1 ☑☐☐☐ **RÈGLE A5** (1ʳᵉ partie)

Je me teste

TEST INTUITIF

Encerclez la forme que <u>vous</u> employez.

▶ En rédigeant, j'écrirais spontanément…

1. a) bas-fond   b) basfond
2. a) bas-relief   b) basrelief
3. a) basse-cour   b) bassecour
4. a) les bien-faits   b) les bienfaits
5. a) le bien-fondé   b) le bienfondé
6. a) haut-commissariat b) hautcommissariat
7. a) haut-parleur   b) hautparleur
8. a) mal famé   b) malfamé
9. a) mal honnête   b) malhonnête
10. a) mille-feuille   b) millefeuille

Quatre formes sont inexistantes. Rayez-les. Le corrigé est à la page 202, et les formes fautives sont signalées à la page 32.

Voyez à l'étape 2 la règle de la soudure avec **bas(se)-**, **bien-**, **haut(e)-**, **mal-** et **mille-**.

consonnes doubles   anomalies rectifiées   choix recommandés

Étape 2 ☑☑☐☐   RÈGLE A5 (1ʳᵉ partie)

Je découvre

NON RECOMMANDÉ	RECOMMANDÉ
une basse-cour	**une bassecour**
le bien-fondé	**le bienfondé**
un haut-parleur	**un hautparleur**
mal famé	**malfamé**
un mille-pattes	**un millepatte**

J'apprends — Soudure

On écrit en un seul mot plusieurs mots composés de **bas(se)-**, **bien-**, **haut(e)-**, **mal-** et **mille-**.

J'ai déjà vu ça — La règle existait en partie

On trouvait déjà des mots tels **un bienfait**, **être bienvenu**, **bienheureux**, **maladroit**, **malchanceux**, **malpoli**, **la malnutrition**, **millefeuille** écrits en un seul mot.

J'observe — Le pluriel se régularise

Ces mots devenus simples suivent la règle générale du singulier et du pluriel. Exemples :
- **une bassecour**, **des bassecours** ;
- **un millepatte**, **des millepattes**.

trait d'union et soudure | singulier et pluriel | accents et tréma

Je fais attention — J'examine les cas

Ce ne sont pas tous les mots qui sont soudés. Il faut bien connaitre chaque cas. Les voici.

Je lis la liste — bas... et basse...

On écrit en un mot uniquement **basfond**, **bassecour** et les mots rares **bassecontre**, **bassecontriste**, **bassecourier**, **bassedanse**, **bassefosse**, **basselice** ou **basselisse**, **basselicier** ou **basselissier**, **bassetaille**.

Je lis la liste — haut... et haute...

On écrit en un mot uniquement **hautfond**, **hautparleur**, **hautefidélité**, **hauteforme** et les mots plus rares **hautecontre**, **hautelice** ou **hautelisse**, **hautelicier** ou **hautelissier**, **hautetaille.**

Je soude — bien...

Plusieurs mots avec **bien-** s'écrivaient déjà en un mot, comme **bienveillant**. On ajoute aussi : **bienaimé**, **un biencuit**, **le bienêtre**, **le bienfondé** et les mots rares **le bienaller**, **le biendire**, **la biendisance**, **biendisant**, **un bienfonds**, **un bienjugé**, **le bienmanger**, **bienpensant**, **bienportant**, **bientenant**, **le bienvieillir**, **le bienvivre**, **bienvoulu**.

---

consonnes doubles   anomalies rectifiées   choix recommandés

Je soude — mal...

Plusieurs mots avec **mal-** s'écrivaient déjà en un seul mot, comme **maladresse**, **maladroitement**, **malaisé**, **malcommode**, **malentendant**, **malformation**, **malhabile**, **malheureux**, **malodorant**, **malpropre**, **maltraiter**...

On ajoute **malaimé**, **malfamé** et les mots rares **le malêtre**, **le maljugé**, **malfaire**, **malportant**, **malvie**, **le malvivre**.

Je soude — mille...

Plusieurs mots avec **mille-** pouvaient déjà s'écrire en un mot ou avec un trait d'union. Il est recommandé de tous les écrire en un mot de nos jours. De plus, on régularise leur singulier lorsque c'est requis. Il s'agit de :

- **un millefeuille** (pâtisserie) ;
- **une millefeuille** (plante) ;
- **une millefleur** ;
- **un millepatte** ;
- **le millepertuis** ;
- **le milleraie**.

Relisez bien les pages 29 et 30 avant de passer à l'étape 3.

trait d'union et soudure | singulier et pluriel | accents et tréma

par Chantal Contant

Étape 3 ☑☑☑☐   **RÈGLE A5** (1ʳᵉ partie)

Je m'exerce

BAS(SE)-, BIEN-, HAUT(E)-, MAL-, MILLE-

Niveau de difficulté : ★★★☆☆

Encerclez la forme recommandée.

▶ Selon la règle, il est préférable d'écrire…

11. a) **des hautes-fidélités** b) **des hautefidélités**

12. a) **des basses-cours** b) **des bassecours**

13. a) **un haut-relief** b) **un hautrelief**

14. a) **ma bien-aimée** b) **ma bienaimée**

15. a) **un mille-pattes** b) **un millepatte**

16. a) **un mal-aimé** b) **un malaimé**

17. a) **le bas-ventre** b) **le basventre**

18. a) **le mille-pertuis** b) **le millepertuis**

19. a) **un bas-fond** b) **un basfond**

20. a) **le bien-être** b) **le bienêtre**

Les réponses sont données à l'étape 4.

Ma note :   /10

consonnes doubles   anomalies rectifiées   choix recommandés

Étape 4 ☑☑☑☑ **RÈGLE A5** (1re partie)

Je corrige

BAS(SE)-, BIEN-, HAUT(E)-, MAL-, MILLE-

Voici le corrigé des pages 27 et 31.

La réponse est **b)** pour tous les numéros sauf 2, 6, 13 et 17 : **basfond, bassecour, les bienfaits, le bienfondé, hautparleur, malfamé, malhonnête, millefeuille, des hautefidélités, des bassecours, ma bienaimée, un millepatte, un malaimé, le millepertuis, un basfond, le bienêtre**.

La réponse est **a)** aux numéros **2**, **6**, **13** et **17** : **bas-relief, haut-commissariat, un haut-relief, le bas-ventre**. Ces mots ne sont pas touchés par la règle A5.

⊗ Les formes données en **4a** et **9a** n'existent pas : on écrit toujours en un seul mot **les bienfaits** et **malhonnête**. Les graphies soudées **2b** et **6b** (dans le test intuitif) de même que **13b** et **17b** (dans l'exercice) sont interdites. Rayez-les.

Vous pouvez réviser les autres formes soudées en relisant les pages 28 à 30.

| trait d'union et soudure | singulier et pluriel | accents et tréma |

par Chantal Contant

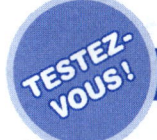

TESTEZ-VOUS !

Étape 1 ☑☐☐☐   RÈGLE A5 (2ᵉ partie)

Je me teste

TEST INTUITIF

Encerclez la forme que <u>vous</u> employez.

▶ En rédigeant, j'écrirais spontanément…

1. a) **un sac fourre-tout** b) **un sac fourretout**
2. a) **des pois mange-tout** b) **des pois mangetouts**
3. a) **un rond-point** b) **un rondpoint**
4. a) **des faire-part** b) **des faireparts**
5. a) **des boute-en-train** b) **des boutentrains**
6. a) **une sage-femme** b) **une sagefemme**
7. a) **un en-tête** b) **un entête**
8. a) **clopin-clopant** b) **clopinclopant**
9. a) **un porc-épic** b) **un porcépic**
10. a) **un terre-plein** b) **un terreplein**

Le corrigé est à la p. 202. Il faut apprendre les formes soudées. L'une de ces formes est inexistante : rayez-la (voyez la p. 40).

Découvrez maintenant à l'étape 2 la règle de la soudure avec **-tout** et les quelques autres soudures ciblées recommandées.

consonnes doubles   anomalies rectifiées   choix recommandés

Étape 2 ☑☑☐☐ RÈGLE A5 (2ᵉ partie)

Je découvre

NON RECOMMANDÉ	RECOMMANDÉ
un **risque-tout**	un **risquetout**
un **sauf-conduit**	un **saufconduit**
prêter **main-forte**	prêter **mainforte**
à **cloche-pied**	à **clochepied**

J'apprends — Soudure

On écrit sans trait d'union les mots composés formés d'un verbe et du mot **tout**.

On soude aussi quelques autres composés bien ciblés. Il faut en connaitre la liste (p. 36).

Je fais attention — Une liste limitée

Ce ne sont pas tous les mots composés qui sont soudés. En effet, les traits d'union ne disparaissent pas tous !

Le Conseil supérieur a recommandé la soudure d'un petit nombre de mots spécifiques : il en a établi une liste limitée. Ce sont surtout des mots dont le sens des composantes n'était plus compris, comme **boute-en-train**, **branle-bas**…

trait d'union et soudure | singulier et pluriel | accents et tréma

Je regarde les exemples ...tout

Les mots composés d'un verbe et de **tout** sont tous soudés. Exemples :

attrapetout	**couvretout**	**passepartout**
avaletout	**essuietout**	**pêchetout**
brisetout	**faitout**	**rangetout**
bruletout	**fourretout**	**risquetout**
cassetout	**mangetout**	**vatout**
coupetout	**mêletout**	

Note : Le pluriel est régulier (ex. : **des fourretouts**).

Je fais le bilan des soudures

Afin de ne pas bouleverser les habitudes d'écriture des francophones et pour éviter de modifier des milliers de mots composés d'un coup, le Conseil supérieur de la langue française a limité les soudures de la règle A5.

En plus des mots touchés par la soudure dans :
— les règles A1 à A4 (p. 11 à 26) ;
— la règle A5, 1re partie, avec **bas(se)-**, **bien-**, **haut(e)-**, **mal-**, **mille-** (p. 28) ;
— la règle A5, 2e partie avec **tout** (ci-dessus) ;
— la règle A5, 3e partie (p. 42) ;
— et la règle G19 (p. 141) ;
les mots ciblés qui doivent dorénavant être soudés (d'après le rapport du Conseil supérieur de la langue française et des travaux de recherche qui ont suivi) apparaissent à la page suivante.

J'observe les soudures ciblées (A5, 2ᵉ partie)

Note : Les mots les plus fréquents ont été cochés. Cochez les autres mots que vous connaissez.

- ☐ ampèreheure
- ☐ arcboutant
- ☐ arcbouter
- ☐ arcdoubleau
- ☑ d'arrachepied
- ☐ boutehors
- ☑ boutentrain
- ☐ bouteselle
- ☐ branlebas
- ☐ chaussepied
- ☐ chaussetrappe
- ☑ chauvesouris
- ☐ chèvrepied
- ☐ clairevoie
- ☐ à clochepied
- ☑ clopinclopant
- ☐ coupecoupe
- ☑ couvrepied
- ☐ crochepied
- ☐ croquemadame
- ☑ croquemonsieur
- ☐ cuissemadame
- ☐ ensoi
- ☑ entête
- ☑ fairepart
- ☐ gagnepetit
- ☐ jeanfoutre
- ☐ jeanfoutrerie
- ☑ mainforte
- ☐ pissefroid
- ☑ potpourri
- ☐ poucepied (crustacé)
- ☐ poursoi
- ☐ poussepousse
- ☐ quotepart
- ☑ rondpoint
- ☑ sagefemme
- ☐ saufconduit
- ☑ terreplein
- ☐ têtebêche
- ☐ triquemadame
- ☐ troumadame
- ☐ vanupied
- ☐ volteface

Ces mots étant maintenant des mots simples, leur singulier devient régulier (**un vanupied**) et leur pluriel également : **des entêtes**, **des rondpoints**, **des sagefemmes**, etc.

trait d'union et soudure | singulier et pluriel | accents et tréma

Après avoir bien regardé tous ces mots, et après avoir pris connaissance des observations ci-dessous à propos de certains d'entre eux, vous pourrez passer à l'étape 3.

Je retiens deux cas — coupe…

Les soudures **coupetout** (haut de la p. 35) et **coupecoupe** (p. 36) relèvent de la règle A5. Les autres composés avec **coupe-** gardent le trait d'union : **coupe-vent**, **coupe-feu**, etc.

Je retiens deux cas — couvre…

Les mots soudés **couvretout** (haut de la p. 35) et **couvrepied** (p. 36) relèvent de la règle A5. Les autres composés avec **couvre-** gardent le trait d'union : **couvre-lit**, **couvre-chef**, etc.

Je soude — croque…

Les formes soudées **croquemonsieur** et **croquemadame** relèvent de la règle A5.

De plus, on trouve dans certains dictionnaires **croquemitaine**, **croquemort**, **croquenote**, **croquethon** en un mot, à côté de la graphie avec trait d'union. La règle G19 recommande alors de choisir, entre les deux formes, celle qui est soudée (p. 141).

Je retiens un cas — gagne...

Le mot **gagnepetit** relève de la règle A5. Par contre, les autres composés avec **gagne-** gardent le trait d'union : **gagne-pain**, etc.

Je retiens huit cas — ...pied

Les huit graphies soudées **d'arrachepied**, **chaussepied**, **chèvrepied**, **à clochepied**, **couvrepied**, **crochepied**, **poucepied** (une sorte de crustacé) et **vanupied** relèvent de la règle A5.

Cependant, les autres mots qui sont composés de **-pied** gardent le trait d'union : **appuie-pied**, **casse-pied**, **gratte-pied**, **protège-pied**, **porte-pied**, **pousse-pied** (petit bateau léger que l'on pousse avec le pied), **passe-pied**, **repose-pied**, **tire-pied**, etc.

Je retiens un cas — pousse...

Le mot **poussepousse** relève de la règle A5. Cependant, les autres mots composés avec **pousse-** conservent leur trait d'union : **pousse-café**, **pousse-mine**, **pousse-pied** (petit bateau léger), etc.

trait d'union et soudure | singulier et pluriel | accents et tréma

Étape 3 ☑☑☑☐ **RÈGLE A5** (2ᵉ partie)

Je m'exerce

SOUDURE AVEC **-TOUT** ET QUELQUES SOUDURES CIBLÉES

Niveau de difficulté : ★★★★☆

Encerclez la forme recommandée.

▶ Selon la règle, il est préférable d'écrire…

11. a) d'arrache-pied   b) d'arrachepied
12. a) pot-pourri   b) potpourri
13. a) un va-nu-pieds   b) un vanupied
14. a) chauve-souris   b) chauvesouris
15. a) un sauf-conduit   b) un saufconduit
16. a) un guet-apens   b) un guetapens
17. a) quote-part   b) quotepart
18. a) des essuie-tout   b) des essuietouts
19. a) faire volte-face   b) faire volteface
20. a) un brise-tout   b) un brisetout

Les réponses sont données à l'étape 4.

Ma note : /10

consonnes doubles   anomalies rectifiées   choix recommandés

Étape 4 ☑☑☑ — RÈGLE A5 (2ᵉ partie)

Je corrige

SOUDURE AVEC **-TOUT** ET QUELQUES SOUDURES CIBLÉES

Voici le corrigé des pages 33 et 39.

La réponse est **b)** pour tous les numéros sauf 9 et 16 : **un sac fourretout**, **des pois mangetouts**, **un rondpoint**, **des faireparts**, **des boutentrains**, **une sagefemme**, **un entête**, **clopinclopant**, **un terreplein**, **d'arrachepied**, **potpourri**, **un vanupied**, **chauvesouris**, **un saufconduit**, **quotepart**, **des essuietouts**, **faire volteface**, **un brisetout**.

La réponse est **a)** aux numéros **9** et **16** : **porc-épic**, **un guet-apens**. Ces mots ne sont pas touchés, car ils ne figurent pas dans la liste du rapport du Conseil supérieur de la langue française.

⊗ La graphie soudée **9b** dans le test et la graphie soudée **16b** dans l'exercice n'existent pas. Rayez-les.

trait d'union et soudure | singulier et pluriel | accents et tréma

TESTEZ-VOUS!

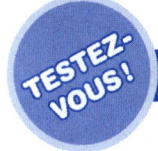

Étape 1 ☑☐☐☐ **A5** (3ᵉ partie) et **G19**

Je me teste

TEST INTUITIF

Encerclez la forme que <u>vous</u> employez.

▶ En rédigeant, j'écrirais spontanément…

1. a) **un pare-brise** b) **un parebrise**
2. a) **un pare-soleil** b) **un paresoleil**
3. a) **un pare-chocs** b) **un parechoc**
4. a) **un pare-avalanches** b) **un paravalanche**
5. a) **un passe-montagne** b) **un passemontagne**
6. a) **un passe-port** b) **un passeport**
7. a) **un porte-feuille** b) **un portefeuille**
8. a) **un porte-monnaie** b) **un portemonnaie**
9. a) **un porte-document** b) **un portedocument**
10. a) **tire-bouchonner** b) **tirebouchonner**

Cinq formes sont inexistantes. Rayez-les. Le corrigé est à la p. 202, et les formes fautives, à la p. 46. Retenez bien les formes soudées.

Découvrez à l'étape 2 quelques soudures avec **pare-**, **passe-**, **porte-** et **tire-**.

---

consonnes doubles — anomalies rectifiées — choix recommandés

Étape 2 ☑☑☐☐ RÈGLES A5 (3ᵉ partie) et G19

Je découvre

NON RECOMMANDÉ	RECOMMANDÉ
un pare-avalanches	**un paravalanche**
tour de passe-passe	**tour de passepasse**
un porte-clés	**un porteclé**
un tire-bouchon	**un tirebouchon**

J'apprends — Soudure

On soude quelques composés bien ciblés avec **pare-**, **passe-**, **porte-** et **tire-**. Il faut bien les connaitre. Il suffit de lire les pages 42 à 44.

Je retiens cinq cas — pare…

On trouve dans des dictionnaires les formes **paravalanche**, **parebrise**, **parebrousaille**, **parechignon**, **parechoc** en un mot, à côté de la forme avec un trait d'union.

La règle G19 recommande alors de choisir, entre les deux, la forme soudée (page 141).

Par contre, les autres mots composés avec **pare-** gardent le trait d'union : **pare-balle**, **pare-boue**, **pare-bruit**, **pare-étincelle**, **pare-feu**, **pare-fumée**, **pare-soleil**, etc.

---

trait d'union et soudure | singulier et pluriel | accents et tréma

Je retiens huit cas   passe...

Les formes **passepartout**, **passepasse** et **passetemps** relèvent de la règle A5. De plus, les dictionnaires donnaient déjà **passerose**, **passavant** (anciennement écrit : passe-avant), **passegris**, **passepoil** et **passeport** en un mot. On les écrit donc soudés.

Cependant, les autres composés avec **passe-** gardent le trait d'union : **passe-montagne**, **passe-carreau**, **passe-droit**, **passe-fil**, etc.

Je retiens onze cas   porte...

La soudure des mots **porteclé**, **portecrayon**, **portemonnaie**, **porteplume** et **portevoix** relève de la règle A5. Les mots **portefeuille** et **portefaix**, eux, étaient déjà soudés.

On trouve dans des dictionnaires **porteballe** (petit mercier), **portefort**, **portemanteau** et **portemine** en un mot, à côté de la forme avec un trait d'union. La règle G19 demande alors de choisir la forme soudée (page 141).

Par contre, les autres composés avec **porte-** gardent le trait d'union. Ils sont nombreux : **porte-aiguille**, **porte-avion**, **porte-balai**, **porte-bagage**, **porte-bébé**, **porte-billet**, **porte-bonheur**, **porte-document**, **porte-drapeau**, **porte-étendard**, **porte-jarretelle**,

porte-parole, **porte-poussière**, etc. Il est inutile de les apprendre par cœur. Retenez seulement les onze cas soudés.

Je retiens cinq cas — tire…

Les mots **tirebouchon**, **tirebouchonnement**, et **à tirelarigot** sont soudés par la règle A5.

Tirebouchonner et **tirefond** relèvent de la règle G19, car on les trouvait déjà en concurrence avec la variante ayant un trait d'union. Il faut choisir la forme en un mot (page 141).

Les autres mots avec **tire-** gardent leur trait d'union : **tire-fesse**, **tire-lait**, **tire-pied**, etc.

J'observe — Singulier et pluriel réguliers

Puisqu'un mot soudé devient un mot simple, il suit la règle générale du singulier et du pluriel. Ex. : **un portecl<u>é</u>**, **des portecl<u>és</u>**.

Je prends une bonne respiration

Vous venez de voir la partie la plus difficile des rectifications de l'orthographe du français : la règle A5 en trois parties, avec la règle G19.

Prenez une bonne respiration, franchissez les étapes 3 et 4, puis détendez-vous : le reste devrait être beaucoup plus facile…

trait d'union et soudure | singulier et pluriel | accents et tréma

par Chantal Contant

Étape 3 ☑☑☑☐   **RÈGLES A5** (3ᵉ partie) et **G19**

Je m'exerce

QUELQUES CAS AVEC **PARE-**, **PASSE-**, **PORTE-**, **TIRE-**

Niveau de difficulté : ★★★★★

Encerclez la forme recommandée.

▶ Selon la règle, il est préférable d'écrire...

11. a) **des passe-droits**   b) **des passedroits**
12. a) **un porte-bonheur**   b) **un portebonheur**
13. a) **un porte-clés**   b) **un porteclé**
14. a) **un gilet pare-balle**   b) **un gilet pareballe**
15. a) **un porte-crayon**   b) **un portecrayon**
16. a) **à tire-larigot**   b) **à tirelarigot**
17. a) **des porte-monnaie**   b) **des portemonnaies**
18. a) **des pare-feux**   b) **des parefeux**
19. a) **un porte-manteau**   b) **un portemanteau**
20. a) **un porte-savon**   b) **un portesavon**

Les réponses sont données à l'étape 4.

Ma note :   /10

consonnes doubles   anomalies rectifiées   choix recommandés

Étape 4 ☑☑☑☑   **RÈGLES A5** (3ᵉ partie) et **G19**

Je corrige

QUELQUES CAS AVEC **PARE-**, **PASSE-**, **PORTE-**, **TIRE-**

Voici le corrigé des pages 41 et 45.

La réponse est **b)** aux numéros **1**, **3**, **4**, **6**, **7**, **8**, **10**, **13**, **15**, **16**, **17** et **19** : **un parebrise, un parechoc, un paravalanche, un passeport, un portefeuille, un portemonnaie, tirebouchonner, un porteclé, un portecrayon, à tirelarigot, des portemonnaies, un portemanteau**.

La réponse est **a)** aux numéros **2**, **5**, **9**, **11**, **12**, **14**, **18** et **20** : **un pare-soleil, un passe-montagne, un porte-document, des passe-droits, un porte-bonheur, un gilet pare-balle, des pare-feux, un porte-savon**. Ces mots ne figurent pas parmi les soudures du Conseil supérieur de la langue française.

⊗ Les graphies **6a** et **7a** n'existent pas : on écrit toujours en un seul mot **passeport** et **portefeuille**. Les graphies soudées **2b**, **5b**, **9b** dans le test et **11b**, **12b**, **14b**, **18b**, **20b** dans l'exercice sont interdites. Rayez-les.

✓ Fin de la règle A5.

trait d'union et soudure   singulier et pluriel   accents et tréma

par Chantal Contant

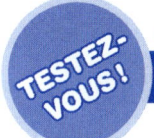

TESTEZ-VOUS!

Étape 1 ☑☐☐☐ RÈGLE A6

Je me teste

TEST INTUITIF

Encerclez la forme que <u>vous</u> employez.

▶ En rédigeant, j'écrirais spontanément...

1. a) cent trente-cinq   b) cent-trente-cinq
2. a) soixante dix-huit   b) soixante-dix-huit
3. a) vingt et un   b) vingt-et-un
4. a) quatre-vingt deux   b) quatre-vingt-deux
5. a) dix sept   b) dix-sept
6. a) dix mille   b) dix-mille
7. a) deux cent quatre   b) deux-cent-quatre
8. a) trente-huit mille   b) trente-huit-mille
9. a) cinq cent mille   b) cinq-cent-mille
10. a) trois millions   b) trois-millions

Avez-vous eu des hésitations ? Comparez vos réponses à celles de la page 203.

Découvrez à l'étape 2 la règle recommandée pour l'écriture des nombres : votre mémoire en sera soulagée.

consonnes doubles   anomalies rectifiées   choix recommandés

Étape 2 ☑☑☐☐ RÈGLE A6

Je découvre

NON RECOMMANDÉ	RECOMMANDÉ
cinquante et un	**cinquante-et-un**
deux cents	**deux-cents**
dix mille vingt-six	**dix-mille-vingt-six**
quatre millions	**quatre-millions**

J'apprends — Trait d'union

Dans un nombre, les éléments d'un numéral composé sont tous reliés par des traits d'union.

J'observe — Aucune exception

Il n'y a pas d'exceptions. On met des traits d'union :
- même autour du mot **et**, comme dans **vingt-et-un** (21) ;
- même si le nombre est supérieur à cent, comme **huit-mille-six-cents** (8 600).

Je sépare deux nombres — Les fractions

Une fraction comprend deux nombres, non reliés. Ex. : **trois-cents dixièmes** (300/10) est différent de **trois-cent-dixième** (310e).

---

trait d'union et soudure | singulier et pluriel | accents et tréma

par Chantal Contant 49

Étape 3 ☑☑☑☐   **RÈGLE A6**

Je m'exerce

TRAITS D'UNION DANS UN NUMÉRAL COMPOSÉ

Niveau de difficulté : ★☆☆☆☆

Encerclez la forme recommandée.

▶ Selon la règle, il est préférable d'écrire…

11. a) cent un   b) cent-un
12. a) deux-mille seize   b) deux-mille-seize
13. a) trente et unième   b) trente-et-unième
14. a) soixante quinze   b) soixante-quinze
15. a) neuf cent trente   b) neuf-cent-trente
16. a) vingt-cinq huitièmes   b) vingt-cinq-huitièmes
17. a) cent quarante-six   b) cent-quarante-six
18. a) quatre vingt dix-sept   b) quatre-vingt-dix-sept
19. a) mille et une nuits   b) mille-et-une nuits
20. a) cent milliards   b) cent-milliards

Les réponses sont données à l'étape 4.

Ma note :   /10

consonnes doubles   anomalies rectifiées   choix recommandés

Étape 4 ☑☑☑☑ RÈGLE A6

Je corrige

TRAITS D'UNION DANS UN NUMÉRAL COMPOSÉ

Voici le corrigé des pages 47 et 49.

La réponse est **b)** pour tous les numéros sauf 16 : **cent-trente-cinq** (135), **soixante-dix-huit** (78), **vingt-et-un** (21), **quatre-vingt-deux** (82), **dix-sept** (17), **dix-mille** (10 000), **deux-cent-quatre** (204), **trente-huit-mille** (38 000), **cinq-cent-mille** (500 000), **trois-millions** (3 000 000), **cent-un** (101), **deux-mille-seize** (2016), **trente-et-unième** (31e), **soixante-quinze** (75), **neuf-cent-trente** (930), **cent-quarante-six** (146), **quatre-vingt-dix-sept** (97), **mille-et-une nuits** (1001 nuits), **cent-milliards**.

La réponse est **a)** au numéro **16** : il s'agit de la fraction **vingt-cinq huitièmes** (25/8).

⊗ Les formes données en **2a**, **4a** et **5a** dans le test intuitif de même que les formes **12a**, **14a**, **18a** et **16b** dans l'exercice n'existent pas. Rayez-les.

✓ Fin de la règle A6.

trait d'union et soudure — singulier et pluriel — accents et tréma

VRAI ou FAUX?

TRAIT D'UNION ET SOUDURE (A1 À A6)

1- En orthographe moderne, tous les traits d'union disparaissent. **V** ou **F**

2- En orthographe moderne, on écrit **contrinterrogatoire** (le **e** de **contre** disparait). **V** ou **F**

3- Par exception, **contre-proposition** conserve son trait d'union pour éviter un mot soudé qui serait trop long. **V** ou **F**

4- On soude le mot **s'entr'accuser** en enlevant l'apostrophe devant le **a**, ce qui donne : **s'entraccuser**. **V** ou **F**

5- On ne peut pas souder **infra-son**, sinon la lettre **s** entre les deux voyelles dans **infrason** se prononcerait « **z** ». **V** ou **F**

6- La graphie **extra-terrestre** avec trait d'union est absente maintenant du *Petit Robert* et du *Petit Larousse*. **V** ou **F**

7- Dans **auto-ironie**, on garde le trait d'union, sinon la soudure provoquerait un problème de prononciation (**oi**). **V** ou **F**

8- Le mot **néo-zélandais** ne doit pas être soudé, car il est en relation avec un nom propre géographique. V ou F

9- On doit maintenir le trait d'union dans **micro-organisme**, pour éviter deux **o** de suite (**oo**). V ou F

10- On conserve les traits d'union dans **oto-rhino-laryngologiste**, pour éviter un mot soudé trop long. V ou F

11- La forme soudée **statuquo** prend un **s** au pluriel : **des statuquos**. V ou F

12- Quand on soude **un mille-pattes**, on enlève le **s** pour rendre le singulier régulier : **un millepatte**. V ou F

13- Certains composés se soudent, tels **sagefemme** ou **potpourri**, comme ce fut le cas jadis pour **vinaigre**, qui est composé de **vin** + **aigre**. Ces mots soudés ont un pluriel régulier. V ou F

14- Selon la règle moderne, le mot **cent** doit être uni par des traits d'union dans un numéral composé, comme dans **deux-cent-trois** (203). V ou F

Réponses à la page suivante

trait d'union et soudure

singulier et pluriel

accents et tréma

RÉPONSES DES PAGES 51 ET 52

1- Faux : seuls les mots construits avec des préfixes ou des éléments savants, les onomatopées, des mots étrangers et quelques autres mots ciblés perdent leur trait d'union.

2- Vrai : **contrinterrogatoire**.

3- Faux : on écrit **contreproposition**. Il n'y a pas d'exception en raison de la longueur.

4- Vrai : **s'entraccuser**.

5- Faux : en frontière de préfixe, la lettre **s** continue de se prononcer « **s** », comme dans **présélection**, **resituer**, **télésérie**.

6- Vrai : seul **extraterrestre** est donné.

7- Vrai : il faut éviter le son « **oi** ».

8- Faux : on soude **néozélandais**. Il ne s'agit pas d'une coordination de deux termes géographiques comme **canado-japonais** (relation Canada-Japon), mais du simple préfixe **néo-** (« nouveau/nouvelle ») devant **zélandais**.

9- Faux : on soude **microorganisme**.

10- Faux : la longueur n'est pas un critère. *Petit Robert* écrit **otorhinolaryngologiste**.

11- Vrai : **des statuquos** (pluriel régulier).

12- Vrai : **un millepatte** (singulier régulier).

13- Vrai : comme **des vinaigres**, on a **des sagefemmes**, **des potpourris**.

14- Vrai : on écrit **deux-cent-trois**.

consonnes doubles — anomalies rectifiées — choix recommandés

Orthographe recommandée : exercices et mots courants

Le singulier et le pluriel

RÈGLES B

trait d'union et soudure | singulier et pluriel | accents et tréma

par Chantal Contant

TESTEZ-VOUS !

Étape 1 ☑☐☐☐ **RÈGLE B1**

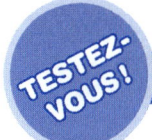

Je me teste

TEST INTUITIF

Encerclez la forme que <u>vous</u> employez.

▶ En rédigeant, j'écrirais spontanément...

1. a) **un lance-flamme** b) **un lance-flammes**
2. a) **un compte-goutte** b) **un compte-gouttes**
3. a) **un rase-motte** b) **un rase-mottes**
4. a) **un sans-papier** b) **un sans-papiers**
5. a) **des grille-pain** b) **des grille-pains**
6. a) **des coupe-vent** b) **des coupe-vents**
7. a) **des casse-tête** b) **des casse-têtes**
8. a) **des sans-abri** b) **des sans-abris**
9. a) **des sous-verre** b) **des sous-verres**
10. a) **des hors-jeu** b) **des hors-jeux**

Regardez les réponses à la page 203, puis découvrez le singulier et le pluriel régularisés.

Au lieu de raisonner sur les deux éléments de ces noms composés, vous aurez simplement à vérifier si c'est **un** ou **des**.

consonnes doubles   anomalies rectifiées   choix recommandés

Étape 2 ☑☒☐☐   RÈGLE B1

Je découvre

NON RECOMMANDÉ	RECOMMANDÉ
un presse-fruits	un presse-frui**t**
un casse-noisettes	un casse-noisett**e**
des brise-glace	des brise-glace**s**
des après-midi	des après-midi**s**

J'apprends — Noms composés

Dans les noms avec trait d'union formés
- ou bien d'un **VERBE** et d'un **NOM COMMUN** (comme *presse-fruit*) ;
- ou bien d'une **PRÉPOSITION** et d'un **NOM COMMUN** (comme *après-midi*) ;

la marque de pluriel est toujours présente sur le second élément uniquement si le mot composé est au pluriel : **un presse-fruit**, **des presse-fruits**.

J'observe — Il y avait des contradictions

Un dictionnaire écrivait *des brise-glaces*, alors qu'un autre écrivait *des brise-glace*… Et un même dictionnaire donnait *un presse-citron*, mais *un presse-fruits*. Il fallait apprendre par cœur tous ces caprices orthographiques.

trait d'union et soudure | **singulier et pluriel** | accents et tréma

Je raisonne autrement — C'est **un** ou **des**

On ne se demande plus si c'est pour presser un ou des fruits, pour briser la ou les glaces.

On applique plutôt le singulier et le pluriel comme on le fait pour les mots simples.

En français, on ne met généralement pas de **s** à un nom simple au singulier : **un navire**. De même, on écrira **un brise-glace** sans **s**. S'il y en a plusieurs, on met un **s** à **des navires**. Alors, on mettra un **s** à **des brise-glaces**.

Note : Ce mot ne désigne d'ailleurs pas de la glace ou des glaces, mais bien un navire ou des navires.

J'examine les catégories — verbe ou prép.

Cette règle s'applique aux composés formés de **VERBE** + **NOM** et de **PRÉPOSITION** + **NOM**.

Elle ne s'applique donc pas aux mots comme *grand-père, arc-en-ciel, laissez-passer*…

Je note — Pas de majuscule, pas d'article

La règle ne s'applique pas si le 2ᵉ élément :
- est un nom propre (avec majuscule, comme dans *prie-Dieu*) ;
- ou contient un article (comme dans *trompe-l'œil, crève-la-faim, sans-le-sou*).

Étape 3 ☑☑☑☐   RÈGLE B1

Je m'exerce

VERBE + NOM : SINGULIER ET PLURIEL RÉGULIERS

Niveau de difficulté : ★☆☆☆☆

Encerclez la forme recommandée.

▶ Selon la règle, il est préférable d'écrire...

11. a) **un taille-crayon**   b) un taille-crayons
12. a) **un garde-côte**   b) un garde-côtes
13. a) **des porte-parole**   b) des porte-paroles
14. a) **un tue-mouche**   b) un tue-mouches
15. a) **des abat-jour**   b) des abat-jours
16. a) **des chauffe-eau**   b) des chauffe-eaux
17. a) **un cure-dent**   b) un cure-dents
18. a) **des rince-bouche**   b) des rince-bouches
19. a) **des gardes-pêche**   b) des garde-pêches
20. a) **des chasse-neige**   b) des chasse-neiges

Avez-vous bien vérifié si c'était **un** ou **des** ? Voyez les réponses à l'étape 4 (p. 60).

Ma note :   /10

trait d'union et soudure | **singulier et pluriel** | accents et tréma

par Chantal Contant

Étape 3 ☑☑☑☐ (suite) — RÈGLE B1

Je m'exerce

PRÉPOSITION + NOM : SINGULIER ET PLURIEL RÉGULIERS

Niveau de difficulté : ★★★☆☆

Encerclez la forme recommandée.

▶ Selon la règle, il est préférable d'écrire…

21. a) des sans-cœur b) des sans-cœurs
22. a) un hors-piste b) un hors-pistes
23. a) des sans-fil b) des sans-fils
24. a) des trompe-la-mort b) des trompe-la-morts
25. a) des après-midi b) des après-midis
26. a) des copier-coller b) des copier-collers
27. a) des grands-parents b) des grand-parents
28. a) des sous-main b) des sous-mains
29. a) des chefs-d'œuvre b) des chef-d'œuvres
30. a) des avant-midi b) des avant-midis

Vérifiez s'il s'agit bien d'une préposition suivie d'un nom. Voyez les réponses à l'étape 4.

Ma note :   /10

consonnes doubles   anomalies rectifiées   choix recommandés

Étape 4 ☑☑☑ — RÈGLE B1

Je corrige

NOMS COMPOSÉS : SINGULIER ET PLURIEL RÉGULIERS

Voici le corrigé des pages 55, 58 et 59.

La réponse est **a)** au singulier (1 à 4, 11, 12, 14, 17, 22) : **un lance-flamme, un compte-goutte, un rase-motte, un sans-papier, un taille-crayon, un garde-côte, un tue-mouche, un cure-dent, un hors-piste**.

La réponse est aussi **a)** aux numéros 24, 26, 27, 29. La règle B1 ne touche pas ces mots. ⊗ Rayez 24b, 26b, 27b, 29b (pluriels fautifs).

La réponse est **b)** au pluriel pour les mots composés de **VERBE** + **NOM** (5, 6, 7, 13, 15, 16, 18, 19, 20) ou **PRÉPOSITION** + **NOM** (8, 9, 10, 21, 23, 25, 28, 30) : **des grille-pains, des coupe-vents, des casse-têtes, des sans-abris, des sous-verres, des hors-jeux, des porte-paroles, des abat-jours, des chauffe-eaux, des rince-bouches, des garde-pêches, des chasse-neiges, des sans-cœurs, des sans-fils, des après-midis, des sous-mains, des avant-midis**.

✓ Fin de la règle B1.

trait d'union et soudure | singulier et pluriel | accents et tréma

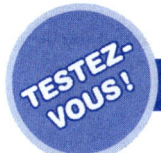

Étape 1 ☑□□□   RÈGLE B2

Je me teste

TESTEZ-VOUS !

TEST INTUITIF

Encerclez la forme que <u>vous</u> employez.

▶ En rédigeant, j'écrirais spontanément…

1. a) **des matches**   b) **des matchs**
2. a) **des ravioli**   b) **des raviolis**
3. a) **des duplicata**   b) **des duplicatas**
4. a) **des conquistadores** b) **des conquistadors**
5. a) **des supernovæ**   b) **des supernovas**
6. a) **des *Pater***   b) **des *Paters***
7. a) **des maxima**   b) **des maximums**
8. a) **des stimuli**   b) **des stimulus**
9. a) **des formats standard** b) **des formats standards**
10. a) **des gentlemen**   b) **des gentlemans**

Avez-vous choisi le pluriel étranger ou bien le pluriel francisé ? Comparez vos réponses à celles du corrigé de la page 203.

Voyez à l'étape 2 la règle du singulier et du pluriel réguliers des mots empruntés.

consonnes doubles   anomalies rectifiées   choix recommandés

Étape 2 ☑☑☐☐   **RÈGLE B2**

Je découvre

NON RECOMMANDÉ	RECOMMANDÉ
des graffiti	des graffiti**s**
des sandwiches	des sandwich**s**
des wallabies	des wallaby**s**
des robes chic	des robes chic**s**

J'apprends — Mots empruntés

Les noms et les adjectifs empruntés à d'autres langues (y compris le latin) suivent la règle générale du singulier et du pluriel des mots français.

J'observe — Singuliers et pluriels

Certains singuliers n'existaient pas et ils ont dû être créés. Ex. : **un varia**, **un zakouski**.

Plusieurs mots étrangers ont deux pluriels dans les dictionnaires. Choisissez le pluriel francisé.

Je note — Prières (rare)

Les noms de prières latines gardent leur valeur de citation (citation du 1er mot de la prière). Ils s'écrivent comme en latin. On les laisse invariables et on les met en italique : des *Pater*.

---

trait d'union et soudure   **singulier et pluriel**   accents et tréma

par Chantal Contant

Étape 3 ☑☑☑☐   **RÈGLE B2**

Je m'exerce

MOTS EMPRUNTÉS : SINGULIER ET PLURIEL RÉGULIERS

Niveau de difficulté : ★☆☆☆☆

Encerclez la forme recommandée.

▶ Selon la règle, il est préférable d'écrire…

11. a) **des cannelloni**   b) **des cannellonis**
12. a) **des gens snob**   b) **des gens snobs**
13. a) **des oméga**   b) **des omégas**
14. a) **des lunches**   b) **des lunchs**
15. a) **des soprani**   b) **des sopranos**
16. a) **des crescendo**   b) **des crescendos**
17. a) **des *requiem***   b) **des *requiems***
18. a) **des chasseurs inuit**   b) **des chasseurs inuits**
19. a) **des paparazzi**   b) **des paparazzis**
20. a) **des varia**   b) **des varias**

Les réponses sont données à l'étape 4.

Ma note :   /10

consonnes doubles   anomalies rectifiées   choix recommandés

Étape 4 ☑☑☑☑   RÈGLE B2

Je corrige

MOTS EMPRUNTÉS : SINGULIER ET PLURIEL RÉGULIERS

Voici le corrigé des pages 61 et 63.

La réponse est **b)** sauf aux numéros 6 et 17 : **des matchs, des raviolis, des duplicatas, des conquistadors, des supernovas, des maximums, des stimulus, des formats standards, des gentlemans, des cannellonis, des gens snobs, des omégas, des lunchs, des sopranos, des crescendos, des chasseurs inuits, des paparazzis, des varias**.

La réponse est **a)** aux numéros **6** et **17**, car il s'agit de mots à valeur de citation (premier mot latin d'une prière).

⊗ La forme invariable **2a** n'existe plus. En effet, de nos jours, les dictionnaires courants donnent à ce mot uniquement un pluriel régulier : **des raviolis**. Les graphies avec **s** aux numéros **6b** et **17b** (noms de prières ayant conservé une valeur de citation) sont interdites. Rayez ces formes inexistantes.

✓ Fin de la règle B2.

trait d'union et soudure   **singulier et pluriel**   *accents et tréma*

VRAI ou FAUX ?

SINGULIER ET PLURIEL (B1 ET B2)

1- Le pluriel de **un gratte-ciel** est
des gratte-ciels.   V ou F

2- En orthographe moderne, on doit
écrire **un ramasse-miettes** avec **s**,
car il s'agit d'un objet pour ramasser
plusieurs miettes.   V ou F

3- On ne peut pas écrire **des rabat-joies** ni **des pare-soleils** avec un **s**,
car il y a de la joie et un seul soleil.   V ou F

4- Le mot **cheval** peut prendre un **s**
maintenant au pluriel.   V ou F

5- Un erratum et **un errata** n'ont
pas le même sens.   V ou F

6- Il n'est plus recommandé d'écrire
le mot **scénario** avec le pluriel
italien savant ou ancien **scenarii**.   V ou F

7- On peut dire et écrire **des minimums**
et **des quantums**, mais aussi parfois
des minimas et **des quantas**.   V ou F

Réponses à la page suivante

consonnes doubles   anomalies rectifiées   choix recommandés

RÉPONSES DE LA PAGE 65

1- Vrai : **des** gratte-ciel**s**. Il s'agit de la règle B1 (mot composé de VERBE + NOM).

2- Faux : **un** ramasse-miette. On ne doit plus se demander si cet objet de nettoyage est fait pour ramasser une ou plusieurs miettes, mais bien s'il y a un ou plusieurs objets. Le raisonnement ne se fait plus sur le second mot, mais sur l'ensemble du composé.

3- Faux : on écrit **des rabat-joies** et **des pare-soleils** puisque c'est écrit **des** devant ces noms composés (règle B1 : VERBE + NOM).

4- Faux : on écrit **des chevaux**. Les rectifications de l'orthographe touchent le pluriel des noms composés (règle B1) et celui des mots étrangers (règle B2). Le mot **cheval** n'est ni l'un ni l'autre. Son pluriel est toujours et uniquement **chevaux**.

5- Vrai : **un erratum** (pluriel : **des erratums**) est une feuille sur laquelle on a indiqué une seule erreur ; **un errata** (pluriel : **des erratas**) est une feuille sur laquelle on a indiqué une liste de plusieurs erreurs.

6- Vrai : on écrit **des scénarios**.

7- Vrai : dans des expressions consacrées, on conservera le pluriel avec **a** (et **s**) : **les minimas sociaux, la théorie des quantas**.

trait d'union et soudure | **singulier et pluriel** | accents et tréma

par Chantal Contant

Exercice récapitulatif 1

Je révise

RÈGLES A (SOUDURE et TRAIT D'UNION)
ET RÈGLES B (SINGULIER et PLURIEL)

Encerclez les formes recommandées et rayez les formes non recommandées.

~~des coupe-feu~~ *(des coupe-feux est encerclé)*
des coupe-feux

des croque-monsieur
des croquemonsieurs

des graffitis
des graffiti

jeu de cachecache
jeu de cache-cache

des sans-gêne
des sans-gênes

à contre-courant
à contrecourant

un weekend
un week-end

psycho-affectif
psychoaffectif

basketball
basket-ball

un compte-gouttes
un compte-goutte

entre-temps
entretemps

six cent vingt-huit
six-cent-vingt-huit

un millefeuille
un mille-feuille

un porte-clés
un porteclé

Les réponses sont données à la page 206.

consonnes doubles   anomalies rectifiées   choix recommandés

Les accents et le tréma

RÈGLES C

par Chantal Contant

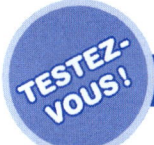

TESTEZ-VOUS!

Étape 1 ☑□□□ **RÈGLE C1** (1re partie)

Je me teste

TEST INTUITIF

Encerclez la forme que <u>vous</u> employez.

Conjugaison : verbe **céder**.

▶ En rédigeant, j'écrirais spontanément…

1. a) **cédant**   b) **cèdant**
2. a) **céde**   b) **cède**
3. a) **cédes**   b) **cèdes**
4. a) **cédent**   b) **cèdent**
5. a) **cédait**   b) **cèdait**
6. a) **cédiez**   b) **cèdiez**
7. a) **cédons**   b) **cèdons**
8. a) **cédera**   b) **cèdera**
9. a) **céderait**   b) **cèderait**
10. a) **céderions** b) **cèderions**

Sept des formes ci-dessus sont inexistantes, donc fautives. Rayez-les. Le corrigé est à la page 203, et les formes fautives, à la page 72.

Retenez la règle de l'emploi du **è** en français présentée à l'étape 2.

consonnes doubles   anomalies rectifiées   choix recommandés

Étape 2 ☑☑☐☐ **RÈGLE C1** (1ʳᵉ partie)

Je découvre

NON RECOMMANDÉ	RECOMMANDÉ
elle cédera	elle c**è**dera
nous céderons	nous c**è**derons
elle céderait	elle c**è**derait

J'apprends — Accent

Au futur et au conditionnel, les verbes comme **céder** changent maintenant le **é** en **è**.

J'observe le son « è » — Un è devant un e

Lever et **céder** se prononcent avec le son « **è** » dans : l**è**ve, l**è**vera, c**è**de, c**è**dera. On écrit donc **è** (et non **é**) avant la syllabe contenant le son « **e** » ou un **e** muet.

Les rectifications de l'orthographe corrigent l'accent aigu fautif au futur et au conditionnel des verbes comme **céder**, afin que la forme conjuguée soit conforme à la prononciation **è**.

J'observe le son « é » — Un é ailleurs

Les verbes comme **céder** gardent le **é** dans les autres contextes : **céd**ons, **céd**iez, **céd**ait…

trait d'union et soudure   singulier et pluriel   **accents et tréma**

par Chantal Contant

Étape 3 ☑☑☑☐   RÈGLE C1 (1re partie)

Je m'exerce

CONJUGAISON DES VERBES COMME **CÉDER**

Niveau de difficulté : ★★☆☆☆

Encerclez la forme recommandée.

▶ Selon la règle, il est préférable d'écrire…

11. a) **je suggére** b) **je suggère**
12. a) **elle suggérerait** b) **elle suggèrerait**
13. a) **nous suggérons** b) **nous suggèrons**
14. a) **ils régleraient** b) **ils règleraient**
15. a) **elles régleront** b) **elles règleront**
16. a) **tu sécheras** b) **tu sècheras**
17. a) **nous tolérerions** b) **nous tolèrerions**
18. a) **vous compléteriez** b) **vous complèteriez**
19. a) **je digérais** b) **je digèrais**
20. a) **je digérerais** b) **je digèrerais**

Pour bien vous aider, repérez d'abord les conjugaisons avec le son « e » ou e muet. Réponses à l'étape 4.

Ma note : /10

consonnes doubles   anomalies rectifiées   choix recommandés

Étape 4 ☑☑☑☑   **RÈGLE C1** (1ʳᵉ partie)

Je corrige

CONJUGAISON DES VERBES COMME **CÉDER**

Voici le corrigé des pages 69 et 71.

La réponse est **b)** avec accent grave lorsque la syllabe qui suit contient le son **e** ou un **e** muet (2, 3, 4, 8, 9, 10, 11, 12, 14, 15, 16, 17, 18, 20) : **cède**, **cèdes**, **cèdent**, **cèdera**, **cèderait**, **cèderions**, **suggère**, **suggèrerait**, **règleraient**, **règleront**, **sècheras**, **tolèrerions**, **complèteriez**, **digèrerais**. C'est un principe général du français, qu'on rencontre aussi dans **crème**, **grève**, **système**, **fidèle**...

La réponse est **a)** avec accent aigu lorsque la syllabe qui suit ne contient pas le son **e** (1, 5, 6, 7, 13, 19) : **cédant**, **cédait**, **cédiez**, **cédons**, **suggérons**, **digérais**.

Les réponses **a)** de 8, 9, 10, 12, 14, 15, 16, 17, 18 et 20 sont les formes traditionnelles du futur et du conditionnel : elles sont non conformes à la prononciation.

⊗ Les réponses **2a**, **3a**, **4a**, **11a** de même que **1b**, **5b**, **6b**, **7b**, **13b** et **19b** n'existent pas en français. Rayez-les.

trait d'union et soudure   singulier et pluriel   **accents et tréma**

par Chantal Contant

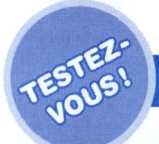

TESTEZ-VOUS !

Étape 1 ☑□□□ **RÈGLE C1** (2ᵉ partie)

Je me teste

TEST INTUITIF

Encerclez la forme que <u>vous</u> employez.

▶ En rédigeant, j'écrirais spontanément…

1. a) **créme**   b) **crème**
2. a) **crémerie**   b) **crèmerie**
3. a) **asséchement**   b) **assèchement**
4. a) **événement**   b) **évènement**
5. a) **dégeler**   b) **dègeler**
6. a) **réglement**   b) **règlement**
7. a) **réglementation** b) **règlementation**
8. a) **élever**   b) **èlever**
9. a) **avénement**   b) **avènement**
10. a) **allégement**   b) **allègement**

Voyez le corrigé, p. 203. Rayez les cinq formes fautives (elles sont signalées à la p. 76.)

Vous découvrirez que d'autres **é** devant **e** sont aussi remplacés par un **è** grâce aux rectifications de l'orthographe.

---

consonnes doubles   anomalies rectifiées   choix recommandés

Étape 2 ☑☑☐☐   RÈGLE C1 (2ᵉ partie)

Je découvre

NON RECOMMANDÉ	RECOMMANDÉ
crémerie	cr**è**merie
événement	év**è**nement
réglementer	r**è**glementer

J'apprends — Un **è** devant un **e**

En général, en français, on écrit **è** (et non **é**) avant une syllabe contenant le son **e**, pour refléter la bonne prononciation. On doit donc remplacer certains **é** incorrects par des **è** devant **e** : s**è**ch**e**resse, c**è**l**e**ri, cr**è**m**e**rie…

Je note — Quelques cas inchangés

Les cas suivants gardent le **é** :
- les préfixes **dé-** et **pré-** (**dégeler**, **prévenir**…) ;
- les **é-** initiaux (**édredon**, **échelon**, **élever**…) ;
- les mots **médecin** et **médecine**.

J'observe — **è** devant -**je** inversé (rare)

Ces cas d'inversions très rares sont rectifiés : **aimè-je**, **eussè-je**, **puissè-je**… (au lieu de **aimé-je**, **eussé-je**, **puissé-je**…), en raison de la présence du **e** muet dans -**je**.

---

trait d'union et soudure   singulier et pluriel   **accents et tréma**

par Chantal Contant

Étape 3 ☑☑☑☐ **RÈGLE C1** (2ᵉ partie)

Je m'exerce

EN GÉNÉRAL, ON ÉCRIT **è** ET NON **é** DEVANT **e**

Niveau de difficulté : ★★☆☆☆

Encerclez la forme recommandée.

▶ Selon la règle, il est préférable d'écrire…

11. a) **réglementaire**   b) **règlementaire**
12. a) **préretraite**   b) **prèretraite**
13. a) **allégrement**   b) **allègrement**
14. a) **céleri**   b) **cèleri**
15. a) **démesure**   b) **dèmesure**
16. a) **sécheresse**   b) **sècheresse**
17. a) **édredon**   b) **èdredon**
18. a) **médecin**   b) **mèdecin**
19. a) **empiétement**   b) **empiètement**
20. a) **pécheresse**   b) **pècheresse**

Avez-vous fait attention aux **é-** initiaux, et aux préfixes **dé-** et **pré-** ? Réponses à l'étape 4.

Ma note :   /10

consonnes doubles   anomalies rectifiées   choix recommandés

Étape 4 ☑☑☑ **RÈGLE C1** (2ᵉ partie)

Je corrige

EN GÉNÉRAL, ON ÉCRIT **è** ET NON **é** DEVANT **e**

Voici le corrigé des pages 73 et 75.

La réponse est **b)** avec accent grave (**è**) aux numéros 1, 2, 3, 4, 6, 7, 9, 10, 11, 13, 14, 16, 19, 20. Notez que la syllabe qui suit contient le son e ou un e muet dans ces mots : **crème**, **crèmerie**, **assèchement**, **évènement**, **règlement**, **règlementation**, **avènement**, **allègement**, **règlementaire**, **allègrement**, **cèleri**, **sècheresse**, **empiètement**, **pècheresse**.

La réponse est **a)** avec accent aigu (**é**) aux numéros 5, 8, 12, 15, 17 et 18, car la prononciation reste **é** dans ces cas (préfixes, **é-** initiaux et *médecin*) : **dégeler**, **élever**, **préretraite**, **démesure**, **édredon**, **médecin**.

Les réponses **a)** de 2, 3, 4, 7, 10, 11, 13, 14, 16, 19, 20 sont non recommandées, car elles sont non conformes à la prononciation.

⊗ Les réponses **1a**, **6a**, **9a** et **5b**, **8b**, **12b**, **15b**, **17b**, **18b** n'existent pas. Rayez-les.

✓ Fin de la règle C1.

trait d'union et soudure | singulier et pluriel | **accents et tréma**

par Chantal Contant

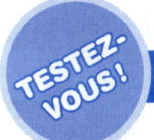

TESTEZ-VOUS !

Étape 1 ☑☐☐☐   **RÈGLE C2**

Je me teste

TEST INTUITIF

Encerclez la forme que <u>vous</u> employez.

▶ En rédigeant, j'écrirais spontanément…

1. a) brûlure   b) brulure
2. a) pupître   b) pupitre
3. a) un fruit mûr   b) un fruit mur
4. a) cîme   b) cime
5. a) assûrément   b) assurément
6. a) je jeûne   b) je jeune
7. a) abîme   b) abime
8. a) bien sûr !   b) bien sur !
9. a) s'il vous plaît b) s'il vous plait
10. a) nous eûmes soif b) nous eumes soif

Comparez vos réponses à celles du corrigé de la page 203. Certaines formes n'existent pas. On vous demandera à la page 82 de les rayer.

Découvrez à l'étape 2 la règle de l'accent circonflexe devenu facultatif sur **i** et **u**.

consonnes doubles   anomalies rectifiées   choix recommandés

Étape 2 ☑☑☐☐   RÈGLE C2

Je découvre

NON RECOMMANDÉ	RECOMMANDÉ
abîme	**abime** (comme **cime**)
chaîne	**chaine** (comme **haine**)
bûche	**buche** (comme **ruche**)
croûte	**croute** (comme **route**)

J'apprends — Accent circonflexe

L'accent circonflexe disparait sur **i** et **u**. Par exemple : **boite**, **ile**, **couter**, **piqure**, etc.

Je note — Un accent distinctif

L'accent circonflexe est maintenu pour sa fonction distinctive dans les cas suivants :

- dans **dû**, **mûr**, **sûr** au masculin singulier ;
- dans **jeûne(s)** ;
- dans les formes du verbe **croitre** qui se confondraient avec celles du verbe **croire** : **crû**, **croîs**, **croît**, **crûs**...

L'accent circonflexe sur ces mots évite de les confondre avec des mots semblables : **du**, **mur**, **sur**, **jeune**, **cru**, **crois**, **croit**, **crus**...

---

trait d'union et soudure   singulier et pluriel   **accents et tréma**

Je note aussi — Des conjugaisons rares

Dans les conjugaisons du passé simple avec **nous** et **vous**, et du subjonctif imparfait avec **il** ou **elle**, on maintient l'accent circonflexe.

Exemples : **nous dormîmes**, **nous eûmes**, **vous finîtes**, **vous fûtes**, **qu'il ouvrît**, **qu'elle bût**.

Cela permet de conserver un parallélisme d'accents dans ces conjugaisons rares (**nous partîmes**, comme **nous arrivâmes**), et de maintenir la distinction entre le subjonctif imparfait (**qu'il fût**) et le passé simple (**il fut**).

Je n'invente pas d'autres exceptions

Les cas présentés ci-dessus et au bas de la page 78 sont les seules exceptions. N'allez pas en inventer d'autres.

La règle s'applique donc bel et bien à des mots comme les suivants :

surement, **sureté**	**une valeur sure**
des endroits surs	**des valeurs sures**
des fruits murs	**une pomme mure**
une mure	**des pommes mures**
jeuner	**il jeunait**, **on jeunera**
croitre	**il croitra**, **on croitrait**
de la bière en fut	etc.

consonnes doubles   anomalies rectifiées   choix recommandés

80 Orthographe recommandée : exercices et mots courants

Étape 3 ☑☑☑☐ RÈGLE C2

Je m'exerce

L'ACCENT CIRCONFLEXE DISPARAIT SUR **i**

Niveau de difficulté : ★☆☆☆☆

Encerclez la forme recommandée.

▶ Selon la règle, il est préférable d'écrire…

11. a) **on connaîtra**   b) **on connaitra**
12. a) **huître**   b) **huitre**
13. a) **nous découvrîmes** b) **nous découvrimes**
14. a) **dîner**   b) **diner**
15. a) **fraîche**   b) **fraiche**
16. a) **un îlot**   b) **un ilot**
17. a) **il apparaît**   b) **il apparait**
18. a) **un gîte**   b) **un gite**
19. a) **il me plaît**   b) **il me plait**
20. a) **un maître**   b) **un maitre**

Les réponses sont données à l'étape 4 (p. 82).

Ma note :   /10

trait d'union et soudure | singulier et pluriel | accents et tréma

par Chantal Contant

Étape 3 ☑☑☑☐ (suite) — RÈGLE C2

Je m'exerce

L'ACCENT CIRCONFLEXE DISPARAIT SUR **u**

Niveau de difficulté : ★★★☆☆

Encerclez la forme recommandée.

▶ Selon la règle, il est préférable d'écrire…

21. a) **une banane mûre**   b) **une banane mure**
22. a) **sûrement**   b) **surement**
23. a) **goût**   b) **gout**
24. a) **nous jeûnerons**   b) **nous jeunerons**
25. a) **il fallut qu'il fût ici** b) **il fallut qu'il fut ici**
26. a) **piqûre**   b) **piqure**
27. a) **du vin en fût**   b) **du vin en fut**
28. a) **un montant dû**   b) **un montant du**
29. a) **des citrons mûrs**   b) **des citrons murs**
30. a) **bûcher**   b) **bucher**

Les réponses sont données à l'étape 4.

Ma note :   /10

consonnes doubles   anomalies rectifiées   choix recommandés

Étape 4 ☑☑☑   RÈGLE C2

Je corrige

L'ACCENT CIRCONFLEXE DISPARAIT SUR **i** ET **u**

Voici le corrigé des pages 77, 80 et 81.

La réponse est **b)** aux numéros 1, 2, 4, 5, 7, 9, 11, 12, 14 à 24, 26, 27, 29, 30 : **brulure, pupitre, cime, assurément, abime, s'il vous plait, on connaitra, huitre, diner, fraiche, un ilot, il apparait, un gite, il me plait, un maitre, une banane mure, surement, gout, nous jeunerons, piqure, du vin en fut, des citrons murs, bucher**.

La réponse est **a)** aux numéros 3, 6, 8, 10, 13, 25, 28 : **un fruit mûr, je jeûne, bien sûr!, nous eûmes soif, nous découvrîmes, il fallut qu'il fût ici, un montant dû**.

⊗ Les réponses **2a, 4a, 5a** de même que **3b, 6b, 8b, 10b, 13b, 25b, 28b** n'existent pas en français. Rayez-les.

On a le droit d'écrire **mûr(e)(s)** et **sûr(e)(s)** avec son accent distinctif si l'on y tient, car les deux orthographes sont admises (détails p. 92).

✓ Fin de la règle C2.

trait d'union et soudure   singulier et pluriel   **accents et tréma**

par Chantal Contant

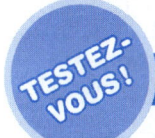

TESTEZ-VOUS !

Étape 1 ☑□□□   **RÈGLE C3**

Je me teste

TEST INTUITIF

Encerclez la forme que <u>vous</u> employez.

▶ En rédigeant, j'écrirais spontanément…

1. a) **un ton aigu**   b) **un ton aïgu**
2. a) **une voix aiguë**   b) **une voix aigüe**
3. a) **elle est naive**   b) **elle est naïve**
4. a) **une notion ambiguë**   b) **une notion ambigüe**
5. a) **désambiguïser**   b) **désambigüiser**
6. a) **de la ciguë**   b) **de la cigüe**
7. a) **exiguïté**   b) **exigüité**
8. a) **des zones contiguës**   b) **des zones contigües**
9. a) **une gageure**   b) **une gageüre**
10. a) **je veux arguer**   b) **je veux argüer**

Deux des formes ci-dessus sont inexistantes, donc fautives. Rayez-les. Le corrigé est à la page 203, et les formes fautives, à la page 86.

Découvrez maintenant à l'étape 2 la règle de l'emploi du tréma.

---

consonnes doubles   anomalies rectifiées   choix recommandés

Étape 2 ☑☑☐☐ — RÈGLE C3

Je découvre

NON RECOMMANDÉ	RECOMMANDÉ
ambiguë	**ambigüe**
ambiguïté	**ambigüité**
gageure	**gageüre**
arguer	**argüer**

J'apprends — Tréma sur u

Les mots qui s'écrivaient avec **-guë-** et **-guï-** s'écrivent maintenant avec le tréma sur le **u**.

De plus, on ajoute un tréma sur le **u** dans **gageüre** et **argüer** (et quelques autres mots rares), pour éviter des erreurs lors de la lecture. Le tréma sur le **u** montre que cette lettre doit être prononcée :
- **gageüre** rime avec **jure** (et non **heure**) ;
- **argüer** rime avec **tuer** (et non **naviguer**).

J'observe — Le tréma sépare deux lettres

Le tréma sert à séparer deux lettres qui formeraient sinon un seul son : **naïf** (évite **ai**), **héroïne** (évite **oi**), **aigüe** (évite le **gu** de **ligue**), **gageüre** (évite le **eu** de **peur**).

---

trait d'union et soudure | singulier et pluriel | **accents et tréma**

par Chantal Contant

Étape 3 ☑☑☑☐   RÈGLE C3

Je m'exerce

TRÉMA DÉPLACÉ OU AJOUTÉ SUR **u** DANS QUELQUES MOTS

Niveau de difficulté : ★★★☆☆

Encerclez la forme recommandée.

▶ Selon la règle, il est préférable d'écrire...

11. a) une note suraiguë   b) une note suraigüe
12. a) la contiguïté   b) la contigüité
13. a) j'argue   b) j'argüe
14. a) des salles exiguës   b) des salles exigües
15. a) des salons exigus   b) des salons exigüs
16. a) une ambiguïté   b) une ambigüité
17. a) la phase subaiguë   b) la phase subaigüe
18. a) nous arguons   b) nous argüons
19. a) deux gageures   b) deux gageüres
20. a) il désambiguïsera   b) il désambigüisera

Les réponses sont données à l'étape 4.

Ma note :   /10

---

consonnes doubles   anomalies rectifiées   choix recommandés

Étape 4 ☑☑☑ RÈGLE C3

Je corrige

TRÉMA DÉPLACÉ OU AJOUTÉ SUR **u** DANS QUELQUES MOTS

Voici le corrigé des pages 83 et 85.

La réponse est **b)** pour tous les numéros sauf 1 et 15 : **une voix aigüe, elle est naïve, une notion ambigüe, désambigüiser, de la cigüe, exigüité, des zones contigües, une gageüre, je veux argüer, une note suraigüe, la contigüité, j'argüe, des salles exigües, une ambigüité, la phase subaigüe, nous argüons, deux gageüres, il désambigüisera**. Cette liste illustre presque tous les changements. Mentionnons, pour la compléter, le déplacement du tréma dans **désambigüisation** et dans les mots rares **bégüe, besaigüe** et **bisaigüe**. Pour l'ajout du tréma, on trouve quelques autres mots en **-geüre** assez rares tels **bringeüre, égrugeüre, mangeüre, renvergeüre**...

La réponse est **a)** aux numéros **1** et **15** : **un ton aigu, des salons exigus**.

⊗ Les formes **1b** et **3a** dans le test et aussi **15b** dans l'exercice n'existent pas. Rayez-les.

✓ Fin de la règle C3.

par Chantal Contant

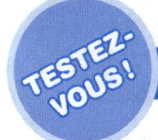

TESTEZ-VOUS!

Étape 1 ☑□□□ RÈGLE C4

Je me teste

TEST INTUITIF

Encerclez la forme que <u>vous</u> employez.

▶ En rédigeant, j'écrirais spontanément…

1. a) **revolver** b) **révolver**
2. a) **scenario** b) **scénario**
3. a) **referendum** b) **référendum**
4. a) **pizzeria** b) **pizzéria**
5. a) **réciter le** *Credo* b) **réciter le** *Crédo*
6. a) **un credo politique** b) **un crédo politique**
7. a) **tremolo** b) **trémolo**
8. a) **cafeteria** b) **cafétéria**
9. a) **media** b) **média**
10. a) **chanter a capella** b) **chanter à capella**

Comparez vos réponses à celles du corrigé de la page 204. Vous employez probablement **déjà** plusieurs graphies francisées.

Découvrez maintenant à l'étape 2 la règle de l'ajout d'accents sur les mots empruntés.

consonnes doubles   anomalies rectifiées   choix recommandés

Étape 2 ☑☑☐☐   RÈGLE C4

Je découvre

NON RECOMMANDÉ	RECOMMANDÉ
allegro	**allégro**
diesel	**diésel**
tequila	**téquila**
juger a priori	**juger à priori**

J'apprends — Accents

On ajoute des accents aux mots étrangers qui en ont besoin pour leur francisation : ces mots doivent suivre les règles françaises.

J'observe — Ils sont nombreux

Les mots empruntés intégrés au français sont nombreux. Voici d'autres exemples de mots accentués : **guérilléro**, **faciès**, **mémento**, **artéfact**, **peppéroni**, **séquoia**, **sombréro**…

Je note — Prières (rare)

Les noms de prières latines gardent leur valeur de citation (citation du 1er mot de la prière). On ne leur ajoute pas d'accent et on les écrit en italique. Ex. : **réciter le *Confiteor***.

---

trait d'union et soudure   singulier et pluriel   **accents et tréma**

par Chantal Contant

Étape 3 ☑☑☑☐   **RÈGLE C4**

Je m'exerce

ACCENTS : MOTS EMPRUNTÉS FRANCISÉS

Niveau de difficulté : ★☆☆☆☆

Encerclez la forme recommandée.

▶ Selon la règle, il est préférable d'écrire...

11. a) **biodiesel**   b) **biodiésel**
12. a) **droit de veto**   b) **droit de véto**
13. a) **chanter un *requiem***   b) **chanter un *réquiem***
14. a) **torero**   b) **toréro**
15. a) **impresario**   b) **imprésario**
16. a) **un joueur senior**   b) **un joueur sénior**
17. a) **a posteriori**   b) **à postériori**
18. a) **un placebo**   b) **un placébo**
19. a) **un gros ego**   b) **un gros égo**
20. a) **jouer moderato**   b) **jouer modérato**

Les réponses sont données à l'étape 4.

Ma note :   /10

consonnes doubles   anomalies rectifiées   choix recommandés

Étape 4 ☑☑☑☑ — RÈGLE C4

Je corrige

ACCENTS : MOTS EMPRUNTÉS FRANCISÉS

Voici le corrigé des pages 87 et 89.

La réponse est **b)** avec accents pour tous les numéros sauf 5 et 13 : **révolver, scénario, référendum, pizzéria, un crédo politique, trémolo, cafétéria, média, chanter à capella, biodiésel, droit de véto, toréro, imprésario, un joueur sénior, à postériori, un placébo, un gros égo, jouer modérato**.

La réponse est **a)** aux numéros **5** et **13** : **réciter le *Credo*, chanter un *requiem***.

⊗ La forme donnée en **7a** n'existe plus. En effet, de nos jours, les dictionnaires écrivent toujours ce mot avec l'accent aigu : **trémolo**. La graphie **5b** dans le test intuitif et la graphie **13b** dans l'exercice n'existent pas (noms de prières latines ayant valeur de citation). Rayez-les. Ne confondez pas la prière (*Credo*) et l'ensemble des principes sur lesquels on fonde sa conduite (un crédo).

✓ Fin de la règle C4.

| trait d'union et soudure | singulier et pluriel | **accents et tréma** |

VRAI ou FAUX ?

ACCENTS ET TRÉMA (C1 À C4)

1- Le verbe **sécher** se conjugue au futur avec un accent grave, comme le verbe **lever** : **il sèchera**, comme **il lèvera**. V ou F

2- Les verbes comme **céder** changent leur accent aigu en accent grave partout dans leur conjugaison. V ou F

3- On doit prononcer « **évènement** », même lorsque l'on écrit **événement**. Il est donc recommandé d'écrire **è**. V ou F

4- Un e dans la syllabe qui suit provoque l'apparition de l'accent grave (**è**) à gauche. On dit et on écrit **réglage**, **réglons**, mais **règle**, **règlementaire**. V ou F

5- Dans **préretraite**, l'élément **pré-** est un préfixe. Il s'écrit avec accent aigu, même si la syllabe qui suit contient **e**. V ou F

6- Dans la phrase littéraire **Je défendrai ces principes, dussè-je y perdre la vie**, on met l'accent grave et non l'accent aigu sur le verbe *devoir* (**dussè-je**), car la syllabe qui suit contient **e** (**-je**). V ou F

consonnes doubles — anomalies rectifiées — choix recommandés

7- L'accent sur **i** et **u** nous obligeait à mémoriser plus de 300 mots ayant un accent difficilement justifiable à notre époque. Par exemple, on devait retenir qu'il y avait un accent dans **épître**, **il plaît**, **voûte**, mais pas dans **chapitre**, **il fait**, **route**. V ou F

8- Toute la conjugaison de **croitre** au futur prend un accent circonflexe pour éviter une confusion avec la conjugaison de **croire**. V ou F

9- Puisqu'il y aurait confusion possible entre les adjectifs féminins **sûre** et **sure** si on enlevait l'accent, on peut maintenir cet accent au sens de « certaine », mais il n'est pas obligatoire de le faire. V ou F

10- Gageure rime avec **heure**. V ou F

11- Avec la nouvelle orthographe, le tréma disparait de certains mots. V ou F

12- Beaucoup de mots sont touchés par la règle du tréma (règle C3). V ou F

13- En français, l'accentuation de mots étrangers tels **trémolo** ou **modérato** a été graduelle. V ou F

Réponses à la page suivante

RÉPONSES DES PAGES 91 ET 92

1- Vrai : on écrit **il sèchera** avec un accent grave (et non un accent aigu) devant **e**, comme dans **il lèvera**.

2- Faux : le **é** se change en **è** seulement devant **e**. Donc, on écrit avec un accent grave uniquement :
- au présent au singulier : **je cède**, **tu cèdes**, **il cède** ;
- au présent au pluriel à la 3ᵉ personne : **ils cèdent** ;
- au futur dans toute la conjugaison (**cèderai**, **cèdera**, **cèderons**...) et au conditionnel (**cèderais**, **cèderait**...) ;

mais pas dans les autres contextes : **cédons**, **cédant**, **cédait**, **céda**, **cédiez**...

3- Vrai : écrire **évènement** est préférable.

4- Vrai.

5- Vrai, car il se prononce toujours « **pré** ».

6- Vrai. Ces inversions avec **-je** sont rares.

7- Vrai. Il fallait les apprendre par coeur.

8- Faux : au futur, par exemple, il n'y pas de confusion possible entre **croitre** et **croire**, car les conjugaisons se prononcent différemment : **elle croitra**/**elle croira**. On n'a donc pas besoin de l'accent circonflexe au futur.

---

consonnes doubles   anomalies rectifiées   choix recommandés

9- Vrai : étant donné que la forme traditionnelle **sûre** et la forme nouvelle **sure** sont toutes les deux admises en français au féminin, vous pouvez choisir de mettre ou non l'accent. Puisque cet accent est utile ici pour distinguer deux sens, certaines instances le recommandent, même si le rapport du Conseil supérieur de la langue française sur les rectifications de l'orthographe insistait sur le masculin singulier seulement. Note : la règle visait déjà le masculin singulier pour **dû/du**.

10- Faux : il rime avec **jure**. L'ajout du tréma évite le problème de lecture, car la présence du tréma sur le **u** dans **gageüre** empêche dorénavant de lire le son « **eu** ».

11- Faux : aucun tréma ne disparait. Le tréma est déplacé dans les suites **-güe-** et **-güi-**, et un tréma apparait dans quelques mots (**argüer**, et mots en **-geüre** comme **gageüre**).

12- Faux : à peine une vingtaine de mots sont touchés par la règle du tréma. La liste presque complète des mots qui sont touchés se trouve à la page 86.

13- Vrai : au fil des siècles, les mots se francisent tranquillement. Certains mots sont déjà pleinement francisés (ex. : **trémolo**), alors que d'autres ont encore deux graphies possibles (avec ou sans accent) dans les dictionnaires.

trait d'union et soudure | singulier et pluriel | **accents et tréma**

par Chantal Contant

Exercice récapitulatif 2

Je révise

Règles C (ACCENTS et TRÉMA)

Encerclez les formes recommandées et rayez les formes non recommandées.

~~elle célèbrera~~ (encerclé : elle célèbrera)
~~elle célébrera~~

juger a priori
juger à priori

dérèglementation
déréglementation

facies
faciès

crèmerie
crémerie

céleri
cèleri

ambiguïté
ambigüité

une voix aigüe
une voix aiguë

un yeti
un yéti

indument
indûment

assèchement
asséchement

un boîtier
un boitier

un client sélect
un client select

ils libèreraient
ils libéreraient

Les réponses sont données à la page 206.

---

consonnes doubles   anomalies rectifiées   choix recommandés

Les consonnes doubles

RÈGLES D

par Chantal Contant

TESTEZ-VOUS !

Étape 1 ☑□□□ RÈGLE D1

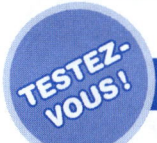

Je me teste

TEST INTUITIF

Encerclez la forme que <u>vous</u> employez.

▶ En rédigeant, j'écrirais spontanément…

1. a) j'appelle un ami   b) j'appèle un ami
2. a) je pelle une pomme   b) je pèle une pomme
3. a) je gelle   b) je gèle
4. a) je chancelle   b) je chancèle
5. a) le morcellement   b) le morcèlement
6. a) le démantellement   b) le démantèlement
7. a) j'époussette   b) j'époussète
8. a) j'achette   b) j'achète
9. a) je jette   b) je jète
10. a) le cliquettement   b) le cliquètement

Comparez vos réponses à celles du corrigé de la page 204.

Découvrez à l'étape 2 la règle qui uniformise l'emploi du **è** (au lieu de la consonne double) devant **e**.

consonnes doubles | anomalies rectifiées | choix recommandés

Étape 2 ☑☑☐☐ RÈGLE D1

Je découvre

NON RECOMMANDÉ	RECOMMANDÉ
il ruisselle	il ruissèle
on renouvelle	on renouvèle
elle cliquette	elle cliquète
ruissellement	ruissèlement
renouvellement	renouvèlement
cliquettement	cliquètement

J'apprends — -èle et -ète

Les verbes en **-eler** et les verbes en **-eter** se conjuguent comme **je gèle** et **j'achète**, c'est-à-dire avec un accent grave devant **e**.

L'accent grave exprime clairement le son « **è** » et remplace l'emploi de la double consonne :
- j'amonc**è**lle devient **j'amoncèle** ;
- il étinc**è**llera devient **il étincèlera**.

J'apprends aussi — -èlement et -ètement

Les noms en **-ement** dérivés de ces verbes prennent aussi l'accent grave : **-èlement** et **-ètement**. Par exemple :
- **amoncellement** devient **amoncèlement** ;
- **étincellement** devient **étincèlement**.

---

trait d'union et soudure | singulier et pluriel | accents et tréma

J'ai déjà vu ça — La règle existait en partie

On avait déjà avec accent grave **je gèle**, **je pèle**, **je modèle**, **j'achète**, **harcèlement**…

J'observe — Il y avait des contradictions

Un dictionnaire écrivait *les poules caquètent*, alors qu'un autre écrivait *elles caquettent*, mais les deux donnaient *caquètement*… La nouvelle règle met fin à ces contradictions.

Je conjugue — présent, futur, conditionnel

Un truc simple : conjuguez ces verbes comme **lever**. L'accent grave apparait devant **e** (donc au futur, au conditionnel, et en partie au présent).

je lève   il lèvera mais **levons   il leva**
je nivèle il nivèlera mais **nivelons   il nivela**

Je note deux exceptions : appelle et jette

Devant **e**, on continue de conjuguer avec une consonne double (plutôt qu'un accent) les verbes **appeler**, **jeter** et leur famille :

j'appelle   mais **nous appelons**
je rappelle   mais **vous rappelez**
il interpellera   mais **il interpela**, etc.

je jette   mais **nous jetions**
je projette   mais **je projetais**
on rejetterait   mais **on rejetait**, etc.

consonnes doubles   anomalies rectifiées   choix recommandés

100 Orthographe recommandée : exercices et mots courants

Étape 3 ☑☑☑☐   RÈGLE D1

Je m'exerce

-ÈLE ET **-ELEMENT**

Niveau de difficulté : ★★☆☆☆

Encerclez la forme recommandée.

▶ Selon la règle, il est préférable d'écrire…

11. a) **tu épelles**   b) **tu épèles**
12. a) **elles dénivellent**   b) **elles dénivèlent**
13. a) **il harcelle**   b) **il harcèle**
14. a) **je rappellerais**   b) **je rappèlerais**
15. a) **ils ensorcelleront**   b) **ils ensorcèleront**
16. a) **un ensorcellement**   b) **un ensorcèlement**
17. a) **un renouvellement**   b) **un renouvèlement**
18. a) **du nivellement**   b) **du nivèlement**
19. a) **le martellement**   b) **le martèlement**
20. a) **le morcellement**   b) **le morcèlement**

Les réponses sont à l'étape 4 (p. 102).

Ma note :   /10

trait d'union et soudure   singulier et pluriel   accents et tréma

Étape 3 ☑☑☑☐ (suite) — RÈGLE D1

Je m'exerce

-ÈTE ET **-ÈTEMENT**

Niveau de difficulté : ★★☆☆☆

Encerclez la forme recommandée.

▶ Selon la règle, il est préférable d'écrire…

21. a) **elle projette**   b) **elle projète**
22. a) **je décachette**   b) **je décachète**
23. a) **on cachettera**   b) **on cachètera**
24. a) **il déchiquette**   b) **il déchiquète**
25. a) **nous rejetterions** b) **nous rejèterions**
26. a) **vous étiquetterez** b) **vous étiquèterez**
27. a) **elles jettent**   b) **elles jètent**
28. a) **on époussetterait** b) **on époussèterait**
29. a) **le cliquettement**   b) **le cliquètement**
30. a) **le craquettement**   b) **le craquètement**

Les réponses sont données à l'étape 4.

Ma note :   /10

consonnes doubles   anomalies rectifiées   choix recommandés

Étape 4 ☑☑☑   RÈGLE D1

Je corrige

-ÈLE/-ÈTE ET **-ELEMENT/-ÈTEMENT**

Voici le corrigé des pages 97, 100 et 101.

La réponse est **b)** avec accent grave pour tous les numéros sauf 1, 9, 14, 21, 25 et 27 : **je pèle une pomme, je gèle, je chancèle, le morcèlement, le démantèlement, j'époussète, j'achète, le cliquètement, tu épèles, elles dénivèlent, il harcèle, ils ensorcèleront, un ensorcèlement, un renouvèlement, du nivèlement, le martèlement, le morcèlement, je décachète, on cachètera, il déchiquète, vous étiquèterez, on époussèterait, le cliquètement, le craquètement.**

La réponse est **a)** aux numéros **1, 9, 14, 21, 25** et **27** : **j'appelle un ami, je jette, je rappellerais, elle projette, nous rejetterions, elles jettent.**

⊗ Les formes **13a** et **19a** n'existent plus : les dictionnaires écrivent **harcèle, martèlement**. La graphie **6a** de même que les graphies **1b, 9b, 14b, 21b, 25b** et **27b** n'existent pas. Rayez-les.

✓ Fin de la règle D1.

---

trait d'union   singulier   accents
et soudure   et pluriel   et tréma

par Chantal Contant

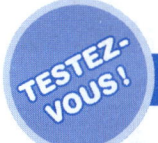

TESTEZ-VOUS!

Étape 1 ☑☐☐☐   **RÈGLE D2**

Je me teste

TEST INTUITIF

Encerclez la forme que <u>vous</u> employez.

▶ En rédigeant, j'écrirais spontanément…

1. a) **une pelle**   b) **une pele**
2. a) **une chandelle**   b) **une chandele**
3. a) **un chandellier**   b) **un chandelier**
4. a) **un atellier**   b) **un atelier**
5. a) **un prunellier**   b) **un prunelier**
6. a) **interpeller**   b) **interpeler**
7. a) **j'interpelle**   b) **j'interpele**
8. a) **nous interpellons**   b) **nous interpelons**
9. a) **un lunettier**   b) **un lunetier**
10. a) **un allumettier**   b) **un allumetier**

Comparez vos réponses à celles du corrigé de la page 204.

À l'étape 2, découvrez comment une **simple** consonne et une **double** consonne influencent la prononciation de la lettre **e** à leur gauche.

consonnes doubles | anomalies rectifiées | choix recommandés

Étape 2 ☑☑☐☐   RÈGLE D2

Je découvre

NON RECOMMANDÉ	RECOMMANDÉ
interpeller	interpeler
dentellier	dentelier
prunellier	prunelier
lunettier (deux prononciations)	lunettier ou lunetier

J'apprends   e + consonne simple = « e »

On simplifie quelques consonnes. Pourquoi ?

Lorsque la lettre **e** est prononcée « e » ou est muette, la consonne qui la suit doit être simple.

Il s'agit d'un principe très général en français, comme dans les mots : **camelot**, **chapelure**, **pelage**, **pelure**, **jeton**, **achetable**...

J'observe   e + consonne double = « è/é »

À l'inverse, quand la consonne est double, la lettre **e** à sa gauche ne peut pas être prononcée « e » ni être muette. On la prononce alors « è » ou « é », même si elle ne porte pas d'accent. C'est un principe très général : **elle**, **bellâtre**, **constellation**, **ellipse**, **pelle**, **pellicule**, **cette**, **toilettage**, **nettoyant**...

trait d'union   singulier   accents
et soudure   et pluriel   et tréma

par Chantal Contant

Étape 3 ☑☑☑☐ **RÈGLE D2**

Je m'exerce

CONSONNE SIMPLE APRÈS LE SON « **e** »

Niveau de difficulté : ★★★★☆

Encerclez la forme recommandée.

▶ Selon la règle, il est préférable d'écrire…

11. a) **interpellait**   b) **interpelait**
12. a) **interpellera**   b) **interpelera**
13. a) **interpellé**   b) **interpelé**
14. a) **interpellions**   b) **interpelions**
15. a) **interpellerions** b) **interpelerions**
16. a) **en interpellant** b) **en interpelant**
17. a) **prunellier**   b) **prunelier**
18. a) **lunettier**   b) **lunetier**
19. a) **dentelle**   b) **dentele**
20. a) **dentellière**   b) **dentelière**

Attention : l'un de ces mots a deux prononciations possibles. Réponses à l'étape 4.

Ma note :   /10

anomalies   choix
rectifiées   recommandés

Étape 4 ☑☑☑☑   RÈGLE D2

Je corrige

CONSONNE SIMPLE APRÈS LE SON « e »

Voici le corrigé des pages 103 et 105.

Les deux réponses **a)** et **b)** sont bonnes aux numéros **9**, **10** et **18**, car il y a deux prononciations possibles : **lunettier** ou **lunetier**, **alumettier** ou **allumetier**. Si on prononce « **e** », on choisit la consonne simple (**b**).

La réponse est **b)** avec la consonne simple aux numéros **3**, **4**, **5**, **6**, **8**, **11**, **13**, **14**, **16**, **17** et **20**, car la prononciation est « **e** » : **un chandelier, un atelier, un prunelier, interpeler, nous interpelons, interpelait, interpelé, interpelions, en interpelant, prunelier, dentelière**. Les formes **a)** de ces numéros ne sont pas conformes à la prononciation et ne sont donc pas recommandées.

La réponse est **a)** avec la consonne double aux numéros **1**, **2**, **7**, **12**, **15** et **19**, étant donné que la prononciation n'est pas « **e** » : **une pelle, une chandelle, j'interpelle, interpellera, interpellerions** et **dentelle**. ⊗ Les formes **b)** de ces numéros n'existent pas. Rayez-les.

✓ Fin de la règle D2.

trait d'union   singulier   accents
et soudure   et pluriel   et tréma

par Chantal Contant

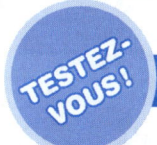

Étape 1 ☑☐☐☐ **RÈGLE D3** (1ʳᵉ partie)

TESTEZ-VOUS !

Je me teste

TEST INTUITIF

Encerclez la forme que <u>vous</u> employez.

▶ En rédigeant, j'écrirais spontanément…

1. a) **écolle**   b) **école**
2. a) **corolle**   b) **corole**
3. a) **bestiolle**   b) **bestiole**
4. a) **moucherolle**   b) **moucherole**
5. a) **fumerolle**   b) **fumerole**
6. a) **barcarolle**   b) **barcarole**
7. a) **babiolle**   b) **babiole**
8. a) **guibolle**   b) **guibole**
9. a) **mariolle**   b) **mariole**
10. a) **colle**   b) **cole**

Voyez les réponses à la page 204. Certaines de ces formes n'existent pas en français. À l'étape 4, on vous demandera de les rayer.

Découvrez à l'étape 2 la règle qui régularise la terminaison des mots en **-ole**.

| consonnes doubles | anomalies rectifiées | choix recommandés |

Étape 2 ☑☑☐☐   RÈGLE D3 (1ʳᵉ partie)

Je découvre

NON RECOMMANDÉ	RECOMMANDÉ
corolle	corole
fumerolle	fumerole
girolle	girole

J'apprends   Mots en -ole

Les mots anciennement en **-olle** s'écrivent maintenant avec une consonne simple : **-ole**.

Les mots de leur famille prennent aussi une consonne simple : **corolaire**, **fumerolien**...

J'observe   Il y avait confusion

On écrivait **école**, **bestiole** et **babiole** avec un seul **l**, mais **corolle**, **moucherolle** et **girolle** avec une consonne double.

Les rectifications mettent fin à cette confusion.

Je note   colle, folle, molle

Les mots **colle**, **folle**, **molle** et leur famille font exception à cette règle. Ils conservent le double **l**.

---

trait d'union   singulier   accents
et soudure   et pluriel   et tréma

par Chantal Contant

Étape 3 ☑☑☑☐   **RÈGLE D3** (1ʳᵉ partie)

Je m'exerce

MOTS EN **-OLE** (ET LEUR FAMILLE)

Niveau de difficulté : ★★☆☆☆

Encerclez la forme recommandée.

▶ Selon la règle, il est préférable d'écrire…

11. a) **girolle**   b) **girole**
12. a) **abeillerolle**   b) **abeillerole**
13. a) **folle**   b) **fole**
14. a) **barquerolle**   b) **barquerole**
15. a) **muserolle**   b) **muserole**
16. a) **arolle**   b) **arole**
17. a) **tartignolle**   b) **tartignole**
18. a) **bouterolle**   b) **bouterole**
19. a) **on décolle**   b) **on décole**
20. a) **corollaire**   b) **corolaire**

Les réponses sont données à l'étape 4.

Ma note :   /10

consonnes doubles   anomalies rectifiées   choix recommandés

Étape 4 ☑☑☑☑   **RÈGLE D3** (1ʳᵉ partie)

Je corrige

MOTS EN **-OLE** (ET LEUR FAMILLE)

Voici le corrigé des pages 107 et 109.

La réponse est **b)** avec la consonne simple pour tous les numéros sauf 10, 13 et 19 : **école, corole, bestiole, moucherole, fumerole, barcarole, babiole, guibole, mariole, girole, abeillerole, barquerole, muserole, arole, tartignole, bouterole, corolaire**.

La réponse est **a)** aux numéros **10**, **13** et **19** : **colle, folle, on décolle**.

⊗ Les formes qui sont données en **1a**, **3a** et **7a** n'existent pas, et les graphies simplifiées **10b**, **13b** et **19b** sont interdites. Rayez-les.

Plusieurs de ces mots sont assez rares. Vous ignorez peut-être le sens de certains d'entre eux. Vous pourrez vous amuser à découvrir la définition de quelques-uns de ces mots grâce au jeu de connaissances (culture générale) à la page 119.

trait d'union   singulier   accents
et soudure   et pluriel   et tréma

par Chantal Contant

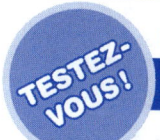

TESTEZ-VOUS!

Étape 1 ☑□□□ **RÈGLE D3** (2ᵉ partie)

Je me teste

TEST INTUITIF

Encerclez la forme que <u>vous</u> employez.

▶ En rédigeant, j'écrirais spontanément…

1. a) **sifflotter**   b) **siffloter**
2. a) **toussotter**   b) **toussoter**
3. a) **frisotter**   b) **frisoter**
4. a) **grelotter**   b) **greloter**
5. a) **neigeotter**   b) **neigeoter**
6. a) **pleuvotter**   b) **pleuvoter**
7. a) **mangeotter**   b) **mangeoter**
8. a) **menotter**   b) **menoter**
9. a) **ballotter**   b) **balloter**
10. a) **nageotter**   b) **nageoter**

Avez-vous trouvé difficile de choisir entre ces graphies ? Voyez les réponses à la page 204.

Découvrez à l'étape 2 la règle qui harmonise la terminaison des verbes en **-oter**.

consonnes doubles | anomalies rectifiées | choix recommandés

Étape 2 ☑☑☐☐ RÈGLE D3 (2ᵉ partie)

Je découvre

NON RECOMMANDÉ	RECOMMANDÉ
frisotter	frisoter
grelotter	greloter
ballotter	balloter

J'apprends — Verbes en -oter

Les verbes anciennement en **-otter** s'écrivent maintenant avec une consonne simple : **-oter**.

Les mots de la même famille prennent aussi une consonne simple : **frisotis**, **grelotement**, **ballotage**…

J'observe — Il y avait incohérence

On écrivait **siffloter** et **toussoter** avec un **t**, mais **frisotter** et **grelotter** avec deux **t**. Il fallait mémoriser chacune des formes.

Je note — menotte, botte…

Les verbes formés à partir d'un nom en **-otte** font exception à cette règle. Ex. : **menotter** vient de **menotte**, **botter** vient de **botte**, alors ils conservent leur double **t**.

trait d'union et soudure   singulier et pluriel   accents et tréma

par Chantal Contant

Étape 3 ☑☑☑☐   RÈGLE D3 (2ᵉ partie)

Je m'exerce

VERBES EN **-OTER** (ET LEUR FAMILLE)

Niveau de difficulté : ★★★☆☆

Encerclez la forme recommandée.

▶ Selon la règle, il est préférable d'écrire…

11. a) **dansotter**   b) **dansoter**
12. a) **garrotter**   b) **garroter**
13. a) **botter**   b) **boter**
14. a) **flotter**   b) **floter**
15. a) **margotter**   b) **margoter**
16. a) **frisottis**   b) **frisotis**
17. a) **ballottement**   b) **ballotement**
18. a) **cachotterie**   b) **cachoterie**
19. a) **cachottière**   b) **cachotière**
20. a) **grelottement**   b) **grelotement**

Les réponses sont données à l'étape 4.

Ma note :   /10

consonnes doubles   anomalies rectifiées   choix recommandés

Étape 4 ☑☑☑☑ **RÈGLE D3** (2ᵉ partie)

Je corrige

VERBES EN **-OTER** (ET LEUR FAMILLE)

Voici le corrigé des pages 111 et 113.

La réponse est **b)** avec consonne simple pour tous les numéros sauf 8, 13 et 14 : **siffloter, toussoter, frisoter, greloter, neigeoter, pleuvoter, mangeoter, balloter, nageoter, dansoter, garroter, margoter, frisotis, ballotement, cachoterie, cachotière** (ces mots sont de la même famille que le verbe rare **cachoter**), **grelotement**.

La réponse est **a)** aux numéros **8**, **13** et **14** : **menotter, botter, flotter**. Ces mots font exception à la règle puisqu'ils sont de la famille de **menotte**, **botte** et **flotte**.

⊗ Les formes données en **1a**, **2a**, **5a**, **6a** et **10a** dans le test intuitif n'existent pas puisqu'on écrit toujours ces verbes avec un seul **t**. À l'inverse, les graphies simplifiées **8b** dans le test de même que **13b** et **14b** dans l'exercice sont interdites. Rayez-les.

✓ Fin de la règle D3.

trait d'union   singulier   accents
et soudure   et pluriel   et tréma

par Chantal Contant

VRAI ou FAUX?

CONSONNES SIMPLES (D1 À D3)

1- Le verbe **renouveler** se conjugue au futur avec un accent grave, comme le verbe **lever** : **il renouvèlera**, comme **il lèvera**.   V ou F

2- Puisque **étiqueter** se conjugue maintenant **j'étiquète** (comme **j'achète**), on mettra aussi un accent sur le nom **une étiquette**.   V ou F

3- Puisque l'on écrit maintenant **un renouvèlement**, on mettra aussi un accent sur l'adverbe **nouvellement**.   V ou F

4- L'arbre qui fournit la cannelle s'écrit avec un seul **l** : **cannelier**.   V ou F

5- Il faut une consonne simple après la lettre e si l'on veut que ce e de gauche soit prononcé « e » (parfois muet).
Ex. : **interpelait, appelait, jetait**.   V ou F

6- Le verbe **bouillotter** vient du nom **bouillotte**. Il doit donc garder deux **t**.   V ou F

Réponses à la page suivante

consonnes doubles   anomalies rectifiées   choix recommandés

RÉPONSES DE LA PAGE 115

1- Vrai : **il renouvèlera**, avec accent grave (et non une consonne double) devant **e**.

2- Faux : seuls les noms en **-ement** dérivés des verbes en **-eler** ou **-eter** sont modifiés pour prendre l'accent grave. On continuera donc d'écrire **une étiquette**.

3- Faux : seuls les noms en **-ement** sont modifiés. Les adverbes ne le sont pas.

L'adverbe **nouvellement** n'est d'ailleurs pas dérivé d'un verbe hypothétique « *nouveler* », mais de l'adjectif **nouveau/nouvelle**, qui est inchangé.

4- Vrai : **cannelle** rime avec **chandelle**, et **cannelier** rime avec **chandelier** et **atelier**.

5- Vrai.

6- Faux : le verbe **bouilloter**, qui signifie « bouillir légèrement », est construit à partir du verbe **bouillir** et du suffixe diminutif **-oter** (qui a le sens de « un peu »). Comme il ne vient pas du nom **bouillotte**, on écrit ce verbe avec un seul **t**.

On trouve le suffixe diminutif **-oter** dans plusieurs autres verbes :

siffloter	nageoter	toussoter
neigeoter	dansoter	mangeoter...

trait d'union et soudure   singulier et pluriel   accents et tréma

Exercice récapitulatif 3

Je révise

RÈGLES A, B, C et D

Encerclez les formes recommandées et rayez les formes non recommandées.

je renouvèle (encerclé)
~~je renouvelle~~

des lave-vaisselle
des lave-vaisselles

il parait
il paraît

corolaire
corollaire

extra-sensoriel
extrasensoriel

une réponse ambigüe
une réponse ambiguë

interpeler
interpeller

événement
évènement

cent cinquante
cent-cinquante

cachotier
cachottier

nivellement
nivèlement

des habits chic
des habits chics

gastroentérite
gastro-entérite

frisotter
frisoter

Les réponses sont données à la page 206.

consonnes doubles — anomalies rectifiées — choix recommandés

✶ Jeu de connaissances
Culture générale I
Je me cultive

Vous avez rencontré beaucoup
de mots jusqu'à maintenant.
En connaissez-vous toujours le sens ?

1. La définition de **foxtrot** est :
a) chien de chasse anglais   **b)** danse américaine

2. Le **statuquo** est :
a) l'ensemble des lois   **b)** l'état actuel des choses

3. Une **sagefemme** est une :
a) femme avisée **b)** spécialiste de l'accouchement

4. Un **tirefond** est un :
a) anneau ou une vis à bois   **b)** cyclone tropical

5. L'expression **à tirelarigot** signifie :
a) à volonté   **b)** de façon improvisée ou bâclée

6. Les **wallabys** sont apparentés aux :
a) cerfs d'Amérique   **b)** kangourous d'Australie

7. Un **crédo** (accentué et en minuscule) est :
a) un carnet   **b)** une prière   **c)** des principes

8. Un **vadémécum** est :
a) un lieu encombré **b)** un aide-mémoire **c)** un vide

9. Le **faciès** est une :
a) expression du visage **b)** frontière fortifiée

trait d'union   singulier   accents
et soudure   et pluriel   et tréma

Consultez un dictionnaire pour en apprendre plus.

Les réponses se trouvent à la page 208.

10. Des **supernovas** sont des :
a) étoiles ayant subi une explosion puissante
b) musiques de danses brésiliennes

11. Une chose est **contigüe** si elle :
a) touche à autre chose   b) est étroite, limitée

12. La **cigüe** est un :
a) insecte mortel   b) poison extrait d'une plante

13. Le verbe **argüer** signifie :
a) se pencher   b) argumenter   c) narguer

14. Un **mariole** est un :
a) malin ou un idiot   b) pantin ou une marionnette

15. Une **guibole** est une :
a) chanterelle   b) jambe   c) offrande ou un don

16. Une **fumerole** est une :
a) émanation d'un volcan   b) tumeur liée au tabac

17. Une **barcarole** est une :
a) chanson de gondolier à Venise   b) petite barque

18. Le verbe **margoter** signifie :
a) comploter   b) voler   c) crier (en parlant de la caille)

Les anomalies rectifiées

RÈGLES E ET F

par Chantal Contant

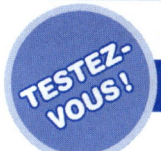

TESTEZ-VOUS !

Étape 1 ☑□□□ RÈGLES E, F1 et F2

Je me teste

TEST INTUITIF

Encerclez la forme que <u>vous</u> employez.

▶ En rédigeant, j'écrirais spontanément…

1. a) **boursouffler**   b) **boursoufler**
2. a) **levreau**   b) **levrault**
3. a) **imbécillité**   b) **imbécilité**
4. a) **asseoir**   b) **assoir**
5. a) **charriot**   b) **chariot**
6. a) **pommiculteur**   b) **pomiculteur**
7. a) **millionnaire**   b) **millionaire**
8. a) **douçâtre**   b) **douceâtre**
9. a) **il est dissous**   b) **il est dissout**
10. a) **on les a laissé fuir** b) **on les a laissés fuir**

Comparez vos réponses à celles du corrigé de la page 204. Deux des graphies ci-dessus sont fautives. Rayez-les (voyez à la page 128).

Découvrez à l'étape 2 des règles qui corrigent des anomalies et harmonisent certains mots.

consonnes doubles | **anomalies rectifiées** | choix recommandés

122 Orthographe recommandée : exercices et mots courants

Étape 2 ☑☑☐☐   **RÈGLES E, F1 et F2**

Je découvre

RÈGLE E : participe passé **laissé**

NON RECOMMANDÉ	RECOMMANDÉ
on les a laissés dormir	**on les a laissé dormir** (comme : **on les a fait dormir**)

RÈGLE F1 : familles harmonisées

NON RECOMMANDÉ	RECOMMANDÉ
bonhomie	**bonhommie** (comme **bonhomme**)
combatif	**combattif** (comme **combattre**)

RÈGLE F2 : séries harmonisées

NON RECOMMANDÉ	RECOMMANDÉ
eczéma	**exéma** (comme **exécuter**)
oignon	**ognon** (comme **rognon** et **grognon**)

trait d'union
et soudure

singulier
et pluriel

accents
et tréma

J'apprends — Anomalies rectifiées

RÈGLE E
Le participe passé du verbe **laisser** suivi d'un verbe à l'infinitif est invariable.

RÈGLE F1
Quelques familles de mots sont harmonisées.

RÈGLE F2
Quelques anomalies sont supprimées, entre autres pour harmoniser certaines séries de mots similaires.

J'observe — laissé + infinitif

Le participe passé de **laisser** se comporte maintenant comme celui de **faire** lorsqu'il est suivi d'un infinitif. Tous deux sont invariables.

- conjugué avec *avoir* :
  Nous les avons fait courir.
  Nous les avons laissé courir.

- en contexte pronominal :
  Elles se sont fait tomber.
  Elles se sont laissé tomber.

La règle d'accord avec **laissé** était hésitante, maintenant elle est claire : on n'accorde pas le participe passé **laissé** s'il est suivi d'un verbe à l'infinitif.

consonnes doubles | **anomalies rectifiées** | choix recommandés

J'observe — Familles et séries harmonisées

L'orthographe française souffre de plusieurs incohérences injustifiées. Le Conseil supérieur de la langue française a décidé d'en corriger quelques-unes, en nombre limité.

Il faut connaitre la liste de ces rectifications.

Elles sont bien ciblées et permettent toutes de rendre plus cohérentes certaines familles ou séries de mots. N'en inventez pas d'autres.

Je lis la liste — Une harmonisation logique

Voici la liste des mots touchés par F1 et F2 :

F1 : familles harmonisées

- ☑ **bonhommie** (comme **homme** et **bonhomme**)
- ☑ **boursouffler** (comme **souffle** et **souffler**)
  boursoufflage, **boursoufflé**
  boursoufflement, **boursoufflure**
- ☑ **charriot** (comme **charrette** et **charrue**)
  charriotage, **charrioter**
- ☑ **combattivité** (comme **battre** et **combattre**)
  combattif, **combattive**
- ☑ **courbattu** (comme **battre** et **battu**)
  combatture, **combatturé**, **combatturer**
- ☑ **imbécilité** (comme **imbécile**)

trait d'union   singulier   accents
et soudure   et pluriel   et tréma

Les mots suivants font aussi partie de la règle F1. Cochez ceux que vous connaissez :

- ☐ **cahutte** (comme **hutte**)
- ☐ **chaussetrappe** (comme **trappe** et soudé)
- ☐ **déciller** (comme **cil** et **ciller**), **décillement**
- ☐ **embattre** (comme **battre**)
- ☐ **innommé** (comme **nommé**), **innommable**
- ☐ **persiffler** (comme **siffler**)
  persifflage, persiffleur, persiffleuse
- ☐ **prudhommie** (comme **homme** et soudé)
  prudhommal, prudhomme (soudé)
- ☐ **sottie** (comme **sottise**)
- ☐ **ventail** (comme **vent**)

F2 : séries harmonisées ou anomalies corrigées

- ☑ **assoir** (comme **j'assois** et **j'assoirai**)
  et sa famille **rassoir, sursoir**…
- ☑ **exéma** (comme **exécuter** et **examen**)
  et sa famille **exémateux**…
- ☑ **nénufar** (on corrige une erreur historique : ce mot vient de l'arabe *nînûfar*, et non du grec)
- ☑ **ognon** (comme **rognon**, **grognon** et **trognon**)
  ognonade, ognonet, ognonière
- ☑ **relai** (comme **balai, remblai, essai** – ces noms ne prennent pas de **s** au singulier : ils sont dérivés de **relayer, balayer, remblayer, essayer**)

Le participe masculin de *absoudre* et celui de *dissoudre* n'étaient pas conformes à la forme au féminin. Les rectifications les corrigent :

- ☑ **absout** (comme son féminin **absoute**)
- ☑ **dissout** (comme son féminin **dissoute**)

L'orthographe posait problème à l'une des prononciations possibles :

- ☑ **ponch** « boisson » – La prononciation de ce mot varie dans la francophonie. On peut écrire **ponch** ou **punch**, selon la prononciation souhaitée.

Les mots suivants font aussi partie de la règle F2. Cochez ceux que vous connaissez :

- ☐ **des appâts** (peu importe le sens)
- ☐ **cuisseau** (peu importe le sens)
- ☐ **douçâtre** (comme **commerçant** et **forçat**)
- ☐ **levreau** (comme **agneau**, **chevreau**, **lionceau**)
- ☐ **saccarine** (on élimine le **h** dans sa famille) **saccarose**, **saccarifier**, **polysaccaride**...
- ☐ **sorgo** (on élimine le **h** dans ce mot)
- ☐ **tocade** (on écrit **c** plutôt que **qu**) **tocante**, **tocard**, **tocarde**

Quand vous aurez bien observé tous ces mots, vous pourrez passer à l'étape 3.

| trait d'union et soudure | singulier et pluriel | accents et tréma |

par Chantal Contant

Étape 3 ☑☑☑☐   RÈGLES E, F1 et F2

Je m'exerce

FAMILLES ET SÉRIES HARMONISÉES

Niveau de difficulté : ★★★★☆

Encerclez la forme recommandée.

▶ Selon la règle, il est préférable d'écrire...

11. a) **combattivité**   b) **combativité**
12. a) **se rasseoir**   b) **se rassoir**
13. a) **relais**   b) **relai**
14. a) **courbatturé**   b) **courbaturé**
15. a) **oignon**   b) **ognon**
16. a) **boursoufflure**   b) **boursouflure**
17. a) **persiffler**   b) **persifler**
18. a) **innommé**   b) **innomé**
19. a) **nénuphar**   b) **nénufar**
20. a) **saccharine**   b) **saccarine**

Les réponses sont données à l'étape 4.

Ma note :   /10

consonnes doubles   **anomalies rectifiées**   choix recommandés

Étape 4 ☑☑☑☑ RÈGLES E, F1 et F2

Je corrige

FAMILLES ET SÉRIES HARMONISÉES

Voici le corrigé des pages 121 et 127.

La réponse est **a)** aux numéros **1**, **2**, **5**, **7**, **8**, **10**, **11**, **14**, **16**, **17** et **18** : **boursouffler, levreau, charriot, millionnaire** (inchangé), **douçâtre, on les a laissé fuir, combattivité, courbatturé, boursoufflure, persiffler, innommé**.

La réponse est **b)** aux numéros **3**, **4**, **6**, **9**, **12**, **13**, **15**, **19** et **20** : **imbécilité, assoir, pomiculteur** (inchangé), **il est dissout, se rassoir, relai, ognon, nénufar, saccarine**.

⊗ Les graphies **6a** et **7b** ne sont pas admises. Rayez-les dans le test intuitif.

Note 1 – Le mot **po**m**iculteur** vient du latin *pomum* « fruit », et non du nom **pomme**. Un pomiculteur (ou pomoculteur) cultive des arbres fruitiers à pépins. Il peut cultiver des poiriers, pas nécessairement des pommiers.

Note 2 – On écrit **millio**n**ième**, mais **millio**nn**aire** : cette famille de mots n'a pas été modifiée.

✓ Fin des règles E, F1 et F2.

---

trait d'union singulier accents
et soudure et pluriel et tréma

par Chantal Contant

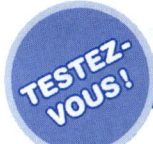

TESTEZ-VOUS!

Étape 1 ☑☐☐☐   **RÈGLES F3 et F4**

Je me teste

TEST INTUITIF

Encerclez la forme que <u>vous</u> employez.

▶ En rédigeant, j'écrirais spontanément…

1. a) **assener** b) **asséner**
2. a) **quincaillier** b) **quincailler**
3. a) **poulaillier** b) **poulailler**
4. a) **québecois** b) **québécois**
5. a) **papeterie** b) **papèterie**
6. a) **féerique** b) **féérique**
7. a) **gelinotte** b) **gélinotte**
8. a) **refréner** b) **réfréner**
9. a) **joaillière** b) **joaillère**
10. a) **marguillier** b) **marguiller**

Note : Deux de ces mots ont deux prononciations possibles. Réponses à la page 204.

Découvrez à l'étape 2 les accents manquants sur quelques mots français et la règle des mots en **-iller** et en **-illère**.

consonnes doubles | **anomalies rectifiées** | choix recommandés

Étape 2 ☑☑☐☐   **RÈGLES F3 et F4**

Je découvre

RÈGLE F3 : accents manquants

NON RECOMMANDÉ	RECOMMANDÉ
assener	**asséner**
refréner	**réfréner**
papeterie (deux prononciations)	**papeterie ou papèterie**

RÈGLE F4 : mots en -iller, -illère

NON RECOMMANDÉ	RECOMMANDÉ
joaillier	**joailler**
quincaillier	**quincailler**

Ces mots riment avec : **conseiller**, **poulailler**

J'apprends   Anomalies rectifiées

RÈGLE F3
Un accent est ajouté dans quelques mots français où il avait été oublié.

RÈGLE F4
Les finales **-illier/-illière** sont remplacées par **-iller/-illère** si le second **i** ne s'entend pas.

---

trait d'union   singulier   accents
et soudure   et pluriel   et tréma

J'observe la règle F3 — Accents manquants

L'accent manquait sur quelques mots français : **asséner**, **réfréner**, **louvèterie**, **gobelèterie**... C'était un oubli, ou bien la prononciation avait changé avec le temps.

J'écoute — Deux prononciations

Deux prononciations sont parfois possibles.

On écrit sans accent ou bien on ajoute l'accent manquant, selon la prononciation souhaitée :

- **féerie** ou **féérie** (au choix) ;
- **vilenie** ou **vilénie** (au choix) ;
- **parqueterie** ou **parquèterie** (au choix) ;
- **gangreneux** ou **gangréneux** (au choix).

J'observe la règle F4 — Prononciation -iller

Joailler rime avec **conseiller** : les deux **l** se prononcent comme dans **fille**. À l'inverse, le mot **millier** n'est pas touché par la règle F4, car on entend le son « l » et le **i** qui suit.

Je note — Arbres et végétaux

Le suffixe **-ier** est maintenu dans les noms d'arbres et d'arbustes comme **groseillier**, **vanillier**, **mancenillier** et **sapotillier**, par analogie avec d'autres noms d'arbres en **-ier** tels **pommier**, **cerisier**, **framboisier**...

consonnes doubles — anomalies rectifiées — choix recommandés

Étape 3 ☑☑☑☐   RÈGLES F3 et F4

Je m'exerce

ACCENTS MANQUANTS ET MOTS EN **-ILLER/-ILLÈRE**

Niveau de difficulté : ★★★★☆

Encerclez la forme recommandée.

▶ Selon la règle, il est préférable d'écrire…

11. a) bougainvillier   b) bougainviller
12. a) quincaillière   b) quincaillère
13. a) marqueterie   b) marquèterie
14. a) un millier   b) un miller
15. a) receleur   b) recéleur
16. a) groseillier   b) groseiller
17. a) cuillerée   b) cuillérée
18. a) papeterie   b) papèterie
19. a) serpillière   b) serpillère
20. a) bijoutier-joaillier   b) bijoutier-joailler

Certains de ces mots ont deux prononciations possibles. Réponses à l'étape 4.

Ma note :   /10

trait d'union   singulier   accents
et soudure   et pluriel   et tréma

Étape 4 ☑☑☑☑   **RÈGLES F3 et F4**

Je corrige

ACCENTS MANQUANTS ET MOTS EN **-ILLER/-ILLÈRE**

Voici le corrigé des pages 129 et 132.

Les deux réponses **a)** et **b)** sont bonnes aux numéros **5**, **6**, **13**, **15**, **17** et **18**, car il y a deux prononciations possibles : **papeterie** ou bien **papèterie**, **féerique** ou **féérique**, **marqueterie** ou **marquèterie**, **receleur** ou **recéleur**, **cuillerée** ou **cuillérée**. Si vous prononcez la lettre **e** comme « **è** » ou « **é** », vous devez mettre l'accent (réponse **b**).

La réponse est **b)** aux numéros **1**, **2**, **3**, **4**, **7**, **8**, **9**, **10**, **12**, **19**, **20** : **asséner**, **quincailler**, **poulailler**, **québécois**, **gélinotte**, **réfréner**, **joaillère**, **marguiller**, **quincaillère**, **serpillère**, **bijoutier-joailler**.

La réponse est **a)** aux numéros **11**, **14** et **16** : **bougainvillier**, **un millier** et **groseillier**. ⊗ Rayez **11b**, **14b**, **16b** (formes interdites).

Note – Un **bougainvillier** rime avec **millier** (et non avec **conseiller**). Comme on entend le **i** qui suit les deux **l**, il n'est pas touché par la règle F4. Cette plante s'appelle aussi parfois **une bougainvillée**.

✓ Fin des règles F3 et F4.

consonnes doubles | **anomalies rectifiées** | choix recommandés

VRAI ou FAUX?

ANOMALIES RECTIFIÉES (E ET F)

1- Grâce aux rectifications de l'orthographe, la règle d'accord des participes passés est grandement simplifiée. **V ou F**

2- On peut maintenant écrire **éléphant** et **pharmacie** avec un **f**. **V ou F**

3- Charriot prend maintenant deux **r**, comme toute la famille des mots construits à partir de **char** : **charrette**, **charrier**, **charrue**, **charroyer**, etc. **V ou F**

4- Les gens sont souvent surpris d'apprendre que l'on peut écrire **ognon** sans **i**. Pourtant, il y a plusieurs siècles, on écrivait avec un **i** les mots **roignon**, **besoigne**, **montaigne**, **lasaigne**, mais on ne le fait plus. Le mot **oignon** est en train de vivre la même évolution. Il a d'ailleurs déjà existé sous sa forme **ognon** dans les dictionnaires d'autrefois. On lui redonne cette forme aujourd'hui. **V ou F**

5- Les règles F corrigent toutes les anomalies dans les familles de mots. **V ou F**

Réponses à la page suivante

---

trait d'union　　singulier　　accents
et soudure　　et pluriel　　et tréma

RÉPONSES DE LA PAGE 134

1- Faux : seul l'accord de **laissé** suivi d'un infinitif a été simplifié. On continue donc d'appliquer la règle traditionnelle aux autres participes passés.

2- Faux : **nénufar** est le seul mot dont le **ph** a été changé en **f**, pour rectifier une erreur historique dans ce mot. Les autres **ph** restent intacts (voyez cependant la règle G16 : si deux orthographes coexistent **déjà** pour un même mot, on doit préférer la forme avec **f** plutôt qu'avec **ph**).

3- Vrai : **charriot** s'harmonise avec sa famille.

4- Vrai : au Moyen Âge, quand le nouveau son « **gn** » a fait son apparition, on le représentait parfois par trois lettres : **ign**, comme dans **seigneur** et **enseignement**. Le **i** après un **a** (**montaigne, lasaigne**) ou un **o** (**roignon, besoigne**) posait un problème de prononciation à la lecture. Ce **i** a donc été enlevé (sauf dans le nom propre **Montaigne**).

5- Faux : elles touchent un nombre très limité de cas (pages 124 à 126). Retenez-les et n'inventez pas d'autres rectifications.

Vous méritez bien une pause détente.

Faites le mot caché qui suit. Il contient des mots des règles D et F, et aussi deux mots des règles G à venir (**iglou** et **mafia**).

consonnes doubles — **anomalies rectifiées** — choix recommandés

★ Jeu — Mot caché

I	M	B	E	C	I	L	I	T	E
N	O	N	G	O	U	B	N	O	R
N	A	A	I	M	A	V	T	I	D
O	A	I	G	B	E	A	E	R	O
M	M	F	L	A	R	S	R	R	U
M	E	A	O	T	V	S	P	A	C
E	X	M	U	T	E	O	E	H	A
R	E	L	A	I	L	I	L	C	T
N	E	N	U	F	A	R	E	O	R
M	I	L	L	E	P	A	T	T	E

Trouvez les mots dans la grille. Il restera cinq lettres.

- **assoir**
- **charriot**
- **combattif**
- **douçâtre**
- **exéma**
- **iglou**
- **imbécilité**
- **innommé**
- **interpelé**
- **levreau**
- **mafia**
- **millepatte**
- **nénufar**
- **ognon**
- **relai**

Réponse (5 lettres) : _ _ _ _ _

trait d'union et soudure   singulier et pluriel   accents et tréma

par Chantal Contant   137

Exercice récapitulatif 4

Je révise

RÈGLES A à F

Encerclez les formes recommandées et rayez les formes non recommandées.

~~des imprésarios~~ (encerclé)   hydroélectricité
~~des impresarii~~   hydro-électricité

relais   en arguant
relai   en argüant

téléenseignement   des égos
télé-enseignement   des ego

réglementaire   revolver
règlementaire   révolver

anti-inflammatoire   des terre-pleins
antiinflammatoire   des terrepleins

un millepatte   une boîte
un mille-pattes   une boite

des vade-mecum   combative
des vadémécums   combattive

Les réponses sont données à la page 207.

---

consonnes   anomalies   choix
doubles   rectifiées   recommandés

138 Orthographe recommandée : exercices et mots courants

Les choix recommandés

Quelle forme choisir
quand deux coexistent déjà ?

RÈGLES G

trait d'union
et soudure

singulier
et pluriel

accents
et tréma

TESTEZ-VOUS!

Étape 1 ☑☐☐☐   **RÈGLES G**

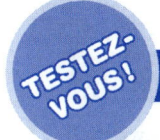

Je me teste

TEST INTUITIF

Encerclez la forme que <u>vous</u> employez.

▶ En rédigeant, j'écrirais spontanément…

1. a) un rockeur   b) un rocker
2. a) une plate-forme   b) une plateforme
3. a) fiord   b) fjord
4. a) la crème antiride   b) la crème antirides
5. a) cacahuète   b) cacahouète
6. a) cannette   b) canette
7. a) estrogène   b) œstrogène
8. a) acuponcture   b) acupuncture
9. a) kleptomane   b) cleptomane
10. a) iglou   b) igloo

Toutes ces graphies existent. Lesquelles sont recommandées ? Réponses à la page 205.

Découvrez à l'étape 2 les règles G. Elles permettent de choisir, quand deux variantes sont en concurrence, celle qui est recommandée.

consonnes doubles   anomalies rectifiées   **choix recommandés**

Étape 2 ☐☑☐☐ RÈGLES G

Je découvre

NON RECOMMANDÉ	RECOMMANDÉ
acupuncture	**acuponcture**
maffia	**mafia**
shampooing	**shampoing**

J'apprends — Choisir la forme recommandée

Si deux formes coexistent, il faut choisir la plus simple ou la plus française (G1-G20). De plus, on suit quatre autres recommandations (G21-G24).

Règle	Variantes	Choix	Exemples
G1	avec acc. circonflexe ou **sans accent**	choisir sans accent	all<u>o</u> nirv<u>a</u>na mihr<u>a</u>b n<u>a</u>gar<u>i</u>
	avec acc. étranger ou **sans accent**		
	avec tréma inutile ou **sans tréma**	sans tréma	<u>i</u>ambique sou<u>i</u>manga
G2	avec h ou **sans h**	sans h	<u>r</u>apsodie
G3	un ou **on**	on	acup<u>on</u>cture
G4	um ou **om**	om	nél<u>om</u>bo
G5	æ ou **é**	é	<u>é</u>gagropile
G6	æ ou **e**	e	<u>e</u>sthésiogène
G7	œ ou **é**	é	ph<u>é</u>nix
G8	œ ou **e**	e	<u>e</u>strogène
G9	u, û, w, oo ou **ou**	ou	cacah<u>ou</u>ète

trait d'union et soudure — singulier et pluriel — accents et tréma

G10	**k**, **kh**, **ch**, **ck**, **cqu** ou **c**	**c**	<u>c</u>leptomane <u>c</u>acatoès
G11	**k**, **ck**, **cqu**, **qu** ou **que**	**qu** ou **que**	ri<u>qu</u>i<u>qu</u>i ja<u>qu</u>ier
G12	**ck**, **ch** ou **k**	**k**	ya<u>k</u>
G13	**sh**, **sch**, **ch** ou **che**	**ch** ou **che**	goula<u>che</u> <u>ch</u>elem
G14	**sch** ou **sh**	**sh**	<u>sh</u>ako
G15	**w** ou **v**	**v**	s<u>v</u>astika
G16	**ph** ou **f**	**f**	para<u>f</u>er
G17	consonne double ou **cons. simple**	**cons. simple**	dri<u>b</u>ler ma<u>f</u>ia
G18	sing./plur. invar. ou **sing./plur. réguliers**	**sing./ plur. régul.**	un antiri<u>de</u> œufs bio<u>s</u> jeux vidéo<u>s</u>
G19	trait d'union ou **soudure**	**soude**	plateforme colvert
G20	complexe ou **simple** étranger ou **français** ambigu ou **non ambigu**	AUTRES CAS : **simple** **français** **non ambigu**	ca<u>n</u>yon cl<u>é</u> pag<u>aille</u> anév<u>ri</u>sme f<u>i</u>ord shamp<u>oi</u>ng granit<u>e</u>
G21	Franciser en **-eur** les finales étrangères des noms en **-er** prononcées « **-eur** » : rockeur		
G22	Tenir compte de certaines innovations reconnues. Ex. : paélia, taliatelle, volapuk…		
G23	Néologisme dérivé d'un nom en **-an** : créer le mot avec un **n** simple. Ex. : gitanologie		
G24	Néologisme dérivé d'un nom en **-on** : créer le mot avec un **n** simple si suivi de **a**, **i** ou **o**. Ex. : fusionite		

consonnes doubles   anomalies rectifiées   **choix recommandés**

J'observe — Deux façons d'écrire

Il n'est pas rare que les dictionnaires donnent deux façons possibles d'écrire un même mot.

Exemple : **clé** ou **clef**. Quelle forme choisir ?

Entre les deux, c'est la forme la plus simple, la plus française, la plus régulière, la moins ambiguë qui est recommandée : **clé**.

Les règles G1 à G20 n'inventent pas de nouvelles graphies : elles ne font que **choisir** entre celles qui existaient déjà.

Je consulte — Comment choisir ?

Comment savoir quelle graphie choisir entre deux ou même trois formes possibles ? Il faut examiner le tableau des règles G (p. 140-141) ou consulter un ouvrage qui contient une liste détaillée de mots avec leur orthographe moderne recommandée (voyez p. 200).

Je retiens quelques autres recommandations

Les règles G21 et G22 sont deux autres recommandations à suivre.

Les règles G23 et G24 s'adressent seulement aux lexicographes et terminologues qui ont à créer de nouveaux mots (néologismes).

trait d'union et soudure   singulier et pluriel   accents et tréma

Étape 3 ☑☑☑☐   RÈGLES G

Je m'exerce

RÈGLES G1 À G4

Niveau de difficulté : ★★☆☆☆

Encerclez la forme recommandée.

▶ Selon la règle, il est préférable de choisir…

11. a) **nirvana**   b) **nirvâna**
12. a) **allô**   b) **allo**
13. a) **emmental**   b) **emmenthal**
14. a) **yogourt**   b) **yoghourt**
15. a) **bizuth**   b) **bizut**
16. a) **néandertalien**   b) **néanderthalien**
17. a) **rhapsodie**   b) **rapsodie**
18. a) **bernard-l'ermite** b) **bernard-l'hermite**
19. a) **acuponcteur**   b) **acupuncteur**
20. a) **columbiforme**   b) **colombiforme**

Toutes ces graphies existent. Il faut choisir la forme recommandée. Réponses à l'étape 4 (p. 149).

Ma note :   /10

consonnes doubles   anomalies rectifiées   **choix recommandés**

Étape 3 ☑☑☑☐ (suite) — RÈGLES G

Je m'exerce

Règles G5 à G9

Niveau de difficulté : ★☆☆☆☆

Encerclez la forme recommandée.

▶ Selon la règle, il est préférable de choisir…

21. a) **présidium**   b) **præsidium**
22. a) **homœopathie**   b) **homéopathie**
23. a) **phénix**   b) **phœnix**
24. a) **œstrogène**   b) **estrogène**
25. a) **gourou**   b) **guru**
26. a) **vroom!**   b) **vroum!**
27. a) **igloo**   b) **iglou**
28. a) **pudding**   b) **pouding**
29. a) **bélouga**   b) **béluga**
30. a) **cacahouète**   b) **cacahuète**

Réponses à l'étape 4 (p. 150). Certaines formes commencent à disparaitre des dictionnaires (ex. : **guru**, **homœopathie**).

Ma note :   /10

trait d'union et soudure   singulier et pluriel   accents et tréma

Étape 3 ☑☑☑☐ (suite)   RÈGLES G

Je m'exerce

RÈGLES G10 À G15

Niveau de difficulté : ★★☆☆☆

Encerclez la forme recommandée.

▶ Selon la règle, il est préférable de choisir…

31. a) **khalife**   b) **calife**
32. a) **caléidoscope**   b) **kaléidoscope**
33. a) **sanscrit**   b) **sanskrit**
34. a) **cleptomanie**   b) **kleptomanie**
35. a) **riquiqui**   b) **rikiki**
36. a) **yack**   b) **yak**
37. a) **chelem**   b) **schelem**
38. a) **haschich**   b) **hachich**
39. a) **shako**   b) **schako**
40. a) **svastika**   b) **swastika**

Toutes ces graphies existent. Il faut choisir la forme recommandée. Réponses à l'étape 4 (p. 150).

Ma note :   /10

consonnes doubles   anomalies rectifiées   **choix recommandés**

Étape 3 ☑☑☑☐ (suite)　　　　RÈGLES G

Je m'exerce

RÈGLES G16 ET G17

Niveau de difficulté : ★★☆☆☆

Encerclez la forme recommandée.

▶ Selon la règle, il est préférable de choisir…

41. a) **parafé**　　　　　b) **paraphé**

42. a) **phlegme**　　　　b) **flegme**

43. a) **téléférage**　　　b) **téléphérage**

44. a) **moufette**　　　　b) **mouffette**

45. a) **canette**　　　　　b) **cannette**

46. a) **maffioso**　　　　b) **mafioso**

47. a) **tanin**　　　　　　b) **tannin**

48. a) **nipponne**　　　　b) **nippone**

49. a) **trimballer**　　　b) **trimbaler**

50. a) **snif !**　　　　　　b) **sniff !**

Toutes ces graphies existent. Il faut choisir la forme recommandée. Réponses à l'étape 4 (p. 150).

Ma note :　/10

trait d'union　　singulier　　accents
et soudure　　et pluriel　　et tréma

Étape 3 ☑☑☑☐ (suite) — RÈGLES G

Je m'exerce

RÈGLES G18 ET G19

Niveau de difficulté : ★★★☆☆

Encerclez la forme recommandée.

▶ Selon la règle, il est préférable de choisir…

51. a) **un anticernes** b) **un anticerne**
52. a) **du pain multigrains** b) **du pain multigrain**
53. a) **des gens sympa** b) **des gens sympas**
54. a) **des produits bios** b) **des produits bio**
55. a) **des jeux vidéos** b) **des jeux vidéo**
56. a) **un électron-volt** b) **un électronvolt**
57. a) **un pique-nique** b) **un piquenique**
58. a) **une plateforme** b) **une plate-forme**
59. a) **des plates-bandes** b) **des platebandes**
60. a) **un fil-de-fériste** b) **un fildefériste**

Réponses à l'étape 4 (p. 150). Pour d'autres exemples de la règle G19, voyez aussi les pages 41 à 46.

Ma note :   /10

consonnes doubles   anomalies rectifiées   **choix recommandés**

148 Orthographe recommandée : exercices et mots courants

Étape 3 ☑☑☑☐ (suite)   RÈGLES G

Je m'exerce

RÈGLES G20 À G22

Niveau de difficulté : ★★☆☆☆

Encerclez la forme recommandée.

▶ Selon la règle, il est préférable de choisir…

61. a) **shampooing**   b) **shampoing**
62. a) **tchao!**   b) **ciao!**
63. a) **guilde** (des musiciens)   b) **ghilde** (des musiciens)
64. a) **semer la pagaye**   b) **semer la pagaille**
65. a) **un interviewer**   b) **un intervieweur**
66. a) **un rockeur**   b) **un rocker**
67. a) **un squatteur**   b) **un squatter**
68. a) **un thriller**   b) **un thrilleur**
69. a) **un sprinteur**   b) **un sprinter**
70. a) **paélia**   b) **paella**

Réponses à l'étape 4. Quand vous rédigez, pensez à choisir la forme recommandée.

Ma note :   /10

trait d'union et soudure   singulier et pluriel   accents et tréma

par Chantal Contant   149

Étape 4 ☑☑☑☑   **RÈGLES G**

Je corrige

RÈGLES G : CHOISIR ENTRE DEUX FORMES EXISTANTES

Voici le corrigé des pages 139 et 143 à 148.

♦ Page 139 – Test intuitif

La réponse est **a)** aux numéros **1**, **3**, **4**, **7**, **8** et **10** : **un rockeur** (règle G21) , **fiord** (G20), **la crème antiride** (G18), **estrogène** (G8), **acuponcture** (G3), **iglou** (G9).

La réponse est **b)** aux numéros **2**, **5**, **6** et **9** : **une plateforme** (G19), **cacahouète** (G9), **canette** (G17), **cleptomane** (G10).

♦ Pages 143 à 148 – Exercices

Les mots dans les exercices apparaissent dans le même ordre que celui des numéros de règles. Les réponses sont parfois **a)** et parfois **b)**.

Il suffit d'appliquer les règles comme indiqué :

♦♦ Page 143 :
11a, 12b, 13a, 14a, 15b, 16a, 17b, 18a, 19a, 20b.
D'abord, la règle **G1** : choisir **sans accent**.
Ensuite, la règle **G2** : choisir **sans h**.
Puis, règles **G3** et **G4** : choisir **on** et **om**.

consonnes doubles — anomalies rectifiées — choix recommandés

♦♦ Page 144 :
21a, 22b, 23a, 24b, 25a, 26b, 27b, 28b, 29a, 30a.
Règles **G5 à G8** : ne **pas** choisir **æ** ni **œ**.
Ensuite, règle **G9** : choisir **ou**.

♦♦ Page 145 :
31b, 32a, 33a, 34a, 35a, 36b, 37a, 38b, 39a, 40a.
D'abord, règles **G10** et **G11** : choisir **c** ou **qu**.
Règle **G12** : choisir **k** (car **c** et **qu** n'existent pas).
Règle **G13** : choisir **ch**.
Règle **G14** : choisir **sh** (car **ch** n'existe pas).
Finalement, règle **G15** : choisir **v**.

♦♦ Page 146 :
41a, 42b, 43a, 44a, 45a, 46b, 47a, 48b, 49b, 50a.
D'abord, règle **G16** : choisir **f**.
Puis, règle **G17** : choisir la **consonne simple**.

♦♦ Page 147 :
51b, 52b, 53b, 54a, 55a, 56b, 57b, 58a, 59b, 60b.
Règle **G18** : choisir le **singulier régulier** ;
choisir le **pluriel régulier**.
Puis, règle **G19** : choisir la **forme soudée**.

♦♦ Page 148 :
61b, 62a, 63a, 64b, 65b, 66a, 67a, 68b, 69a, 70a.
Règle **G20** : choisir la graphie la **plus simple** ou la **plus française**.
Règle **G21** : **franciser** la finale en **-eur**.
Règle **G22** : tenir compte de certaines innovations reconnues.

✓ Fin des règles G.

trait d'union singulier accents
et soudure et pluriel et tréma

VRAI ou *FAUX?*

LES CHOIX RECOMMANDÉS (RÈGLES G)

1- Puisqu'on écrit **allô** ou **allo**, on peut écrire aussi le mot **impôt** sans accent. **V** ou **F**

2- Le mot **théâtre** garde son **h**. **V** ou **F**

3- La graphie **phœnix** a notamment le sens de « oiseau fabuleux qui renait de ses cendres ». **V** ou **F**

4- Puisqu'on peut écrire **iglou** au lieu de **igloo**, on peut conséquemment remplacer le double **o** de **football** par **ou** aussi. **V** ou **F**

5- Puisqu'on a le droit de remplacer **kaléidoscope** et **kleptomane** par **caléidoscope** et **cleptomane** (règle G10), on peut se permettre alors d'écrire aussi **kangourou** avec un **c**. **V** ou **F**

6- La règle G16 permet de remplacer les **ph** par des **f** dans **philosophie**. **V** ou **F**

7- La nouvelle orthographe ne recommande pas l'emploi d'anglicismes, même si les règles G (et B2 et C4) s'appliquent à certains mots étrangers. **V** ou **F**

Réponses à la page suivante

RÉPONSES DE LA PAGE 151

1- Faux : si la forme **allo** est recommandée, c'est parce que cette graphie coexistait déjà, en concurrence avec **allô**. Ce n'est pas le cas pour **impôt** : il n'a qu'une façon de s'écrire.

La règle G1 ne fait pas tomber les accents circonflexes sur les **o**, mais elle recommande de choisir la forme sans accent s'il y a **déjà** deux orthographes pour un même mot dans les dictionnaires. C'est le cas de **allo**.

2- Vrai. La règle G2 ne fait pas disparaitre les **h**. Elle recommande seulement de choisir la graphie sans **h** quand elle existe déjà. Or, le mot **théâtre** n'existe pas sans **h** dans les dictionnaires, contrairement à **r(h)apsodie**, **(h)ululer** ou **yog(h)ourt**, qui ont deux orthographes. **Théâtre** conserve donc son **h**.

3- Faux. La graphie **phœnix** avec œ désigne uniquement une sorte de palmier. Même avant la mise en place des rectifications de l'orthographe, l'oiseau mythologique fabuleux qui renait de ses cendres s'écrivait toujours **phénix** en français (mais pas en anglais). Vous pouvez le vérifier dans un dictionnaire. Attention, ce mot a trois sens : vérifiez bien l'orthographe permise pour chacun.

Comme les botanistes avaient le choix d'écrire **phénix** ou **phœnix** (pour le palmier), la règle G7 leur recommande de choisir **phénix**. Les autres sens s'écrivent toujours **é**.

> **4- Faux** : la forme **iglou** est recommandée, car cette graphie existait déjà dans les dictionnaires, en concurrence avec **igloo** (règle G9).
>
> Les règles G ne demandent pas de remplacer des lettres par d'autres. Elles recommandent de **choisir** la forme la plus simple ou la plus française lorsque deux graphies coexistent **déjà** pour un même mot. C'est le cas de **iglou**, mais pas de **football**.
>
> **5- Faux** : mêmes raisons que ci-dessus.
>
> **6- Faux** : mêmes raisons que ci-dessus.
>
> **7- Vrai**. Les règles vous disent **comment** orthographier tel mot si vous voulez l'utiliser, mais le **choix** du **vocabulaire employé** dans vos textes relèvera toujours de vos décisions.

Avant de tout réviser et de vous soumettre ensuite à une dictée et à l'examen final, vous méritez une pause Dictomanie pour vous amuser.

Ce jeu entremêle astucieusement le principe des mots croisés et celui des mots cachés : d'abord, on trouve la réponse à une question de connaissances, puis on va à sa recherche dans une grille de lettres.

Toutes les réponses du Dictomanie des pages 154 à 158 ont été mises en ligne à l'adresse suivante : www.nouvelleorthographe.info/corrige.html. Pour d'autres jeux Dictomanie sur toutes sortes de sujets amusants, visitez www.dictomanie.com.

consonnes doubles | anomalies rectifiées | **choix recommandés**

154 Orthographe recommandée : exercices et mots courants

★ Jeu — **Dictomanie**

S	E	R	I	O	M	E	M	E	D	I	A	S	E	D	U
N	L	U	O	S	M	U	C	E	M	E	D	A	V	N	N
R	S	H	C	I	W	D	N	A	S	O	C	R	M	U	C
E	E	L	E	V	I	N	O	N	G	O	E	I	E	V	O
I	S	I	L	O	I	V	A	R	M	L	L	U	S	E	M
T	M	A	T	C	H	S	U	B	F	L	Q	I	A	E	P
E	S	A	V	O	N	E	A	F	E	A	U	A	T	T	T
N	O	N	G	O	T	T	U	P	T	A	I	L	O	I	E
U	L	L	A	T	T	O	A	T	E	E	N	E	I	L	G
L	O	H	A	I	S	T	A	R	R	T	C	R	G	I	O
H	C	U	V	R	T	R	V	E	N	T	A	I	L	C	U
T	Q	I	U	E	T	E	G	O	S	O	I	O	O	E	T
S	T	O	X	N	L	A	D	Y	S	G	L	S	U	B	T
E	B	E	O	R	A	R	E	U	G	E	L	S	A	M	E
P	M	C	S	M	U	M	I	N	I	M	E	A	H	I	E
A	C	U	R	E	D	E	N	T	O	I	R	R	A	H	C

Répondez aux questions des pages suivantes en employant la graphie recommandée. Puis, trouvez ces mots dans la grille (sens horizontal/vertical/diagonal).

Réponse :   _ _ _ _ _ _ _ _
(19 lettres)
                _ _ _ _ _ _ _ _ _ _ _

trait d'union   singulier   accents
et soudure   et pluriel   et tréma

L'infinitif du verbe **il assoit** est maintenant :
a _ _ _ _ _

Souffler est de la même famille que le verbe :
b _ _ **r** _ _ _ _ _ _ _

Une **charrue** est de la même famille qu'un :
c _ _ _ _ _ _ **t**

Combattre est de la même famille que le nom :
c _ _ _ _ _ _ _ _ _ **é**

Il attaque, puis j'attaque à mon tour. Donc, **je** :
c _ _ **t** _ _ _ _ _ _ _

Au pluriel, on écrit **des cure-dents** avec un **s**.
Au singulier, on écrit **un** :
c _ _ _ **- d** _ _ _

Au singulier, on écrit **un aide-mémoire**. Au pluriel, on écrit : **d** _ _   **a** _ _ _ **-
m** _ _ _ _ _ _

Certains égoïstes ont un gros **égo**. Au pluriel, on écrira **des** :
é _ _ _

J'ai une maladie de la peau qui la rend fragile ou qui cause des démangeaisons. En orthographe recommandée, on écrira que je suis atteint d' :
e _ _ _ _

156 Orthographe recommandée : exercices et mots courants

Avec de la neige, un Inuit peut construire un :
i _ _ _ _

Un **imbécile** souffre d' :
i _ **b** _ _ _ _ _ _ _

Au singulier, on a **un iota**. Au pluriel, on a **des** :
i _ _ _ _

On a **un gentleman**, **des gentlemans** (pluriel régularisé en français). On a aussi de façon régulière **une lady**, **des** :
l _ _ _ _

On écrit **baleineau**, **renardeau**, **chevreau**, **agneau**... Le petit du lièvre s'écrit maintenant :
l _ **v** _ _ _ _

Léguer prend l'accent aigu à l'infinitif. Par contre, il prend l'accent grave à l'indicatif futur simple. **Il** :
l _ _ _ _ _ **a**

Selon la prononciation souhaitée, on choisit d'écrire **lunettier** ou :
l _ _ _ _ _ _ _

Le pluriel français de **match** s'écrit **des** :
m _ _ _ _ _

Le pluriel français de **minimum** s'écrit **des** :
m _ _ _ _ _ _ _

trait d'union et soudure singulier et pluriel accents et tréma

Geler se conjugue **je gèle** (verbe en **-eler**). Et **niveler** peut aussi se conjuguer ainsi. **Je** :
n __ __ __ __ __

Une nova (et **une supernova**) s'écrivait au pluriel des novæ (pluriel latin). En français, on peut maintenant écrire de façon régulière **des** :
n __ __ __ __ __

Le mot oignon s'écrivait de façon plus simple et surtout plus naturelle avant 1878. On l'écrivait simplement comme **rognon** et **grognon**, donc :
o __ __ __ __
En orthographe moderne recommandée, il est permis de recommencer à écrire oignon sans son **i** superflu, comme avant 1878, c'est-à-dire :
o __ __ __ __
(Ce mot apparait bien deux fois dans la grille.)

Celui qui s'occupe d'une quincaillerie est un :
q __ __ __ __ __ __ __ __ __ __

En italien, le mot pluriel **ravioli** s'écrit sans **s**. En français, par contre, on écrit **des** :
r __ __ __ __ __ __ __

Balayer donne le nom **balai**, et **essayer** donne le nom **essai**. Logiquement, **relayer** donne le nom :
r __ __ __ __ __

Le pluriel français de **sandwich** s'écrit **des** :
s __ __ __ __ __ __ __ __ __

On pouvait écrire **saoul** ou **soûl** (au sens de « ivre »). En orthographe rectifiée, on fait disparaitre l'accent circonflexe sur **u** :
s __ __ __

L'orthographe francisée de **un squatter** est **un** :
s __ __ __ t __ __ __ __

En italien, on écrit **ciao** pour « au revoir ». En français, on écrit de façon moins ambigüe :
t __ h __ __

On écrit **des compte-gouttes** au pluriel. Au singulier, on écrit :
u __ c __ __ __ __ __ -g __ __ __ __ __

On écrivait **un mille-pattes**. De nos jours, on peut l'écrire en un mot et sans **s** (comme **un millefeuille**). Donc :
u __ m __ __ __ __ __ __ __ __ __

Du latin *vade mecum*, qui signifie « viens avec moi », le petit livre que l'on a sous la main et servant d'aide-mémoire s'écrit en français (avec accents aigus et sans espace ni trait d'union) **un** :
v __ __ __ __ __ __ __ __

Le panneau mobile d'une porte (le battant) qui pivote et qui peut être poussé par le **vent** s'écrit en nouvelle orthographe **un** :
v __ __ t __ __ l

trait d'union et soudure — singulier et pluriel — accents et tréma

par Chantal Contant

Exercice récapitulatif 5

Je révise

RÈGLES G

Encerclez les formes recommandées et rayez les formes non recommandées.

~~un complexe multisalle~~ (encerclé)
~~un complexe multisalles~~

yukonais
yukonnais

des appareils monobloc
des appareils monoblocs

téléphérique
téléférique

granit
granite

une réunion intergroupe
une réunion intergroupes

fjord
fiord

cuiller
cuillère

nirvana
nirvâna

dribler
dribbler

emmenthal
emmental

plateforme
plate-forme

cañon
canyon

tanin
tannin

Les réponses sont données à la page 207.

consonnes doubles — anomalies rectifiées — choix recommandés

★ Jeu de connaissances
CULTURE GÉNÉRALE II
Je me cultive

Vous avez rencontré beaucoup
de mots dans ce livre.
En connaissez-vous toujours le sens ?

1. Le mot **tocade** est synonyme de :
a) caprice   **b)** insigne   **c)** femme incapable

2. Le caractère de la **bonhommie** consiste à :
a) être simple et aimable   **b)** faire peur aux enfants

3. La **saccarine** s'apparente :
a) à la caféine   **b)** à la morphine   **c)** au sucre

4. Une **gélinotte** ressemble plutôt à une :
a) coiffe   **b)** perdrix   **c)** cacahouète   **d)** écervelée

5. Une **chaussetrappe** est un :
a) piège   **b)** cordage   **c)** vêtement du Moyen Âge

6. Semer la pagaille signifie :
a) aller aux champs   **b)** créer un désordre

7. Chanter à capella signifie :
a) sans micro   **b)** sans musique   **c)** à tue-tête

8. L'adjectif **nippone** signifie :
a) du Japon   **b)** espiègle et vive   **c)** grivoise

9. Les **taliatelles** sont des pâtes alimentaires :
a) courtes   **b)** en spirales   **c)** longues et minces

trait d'union   singulier   accents
et soudure   et pluriel   et tréma

Consultez un dictionnaire pour en apprendre plus.

Les réponses se trouvent à la page 208.

Associez les mots et les définitions.

10. Associez **yéti** et **yak** à leur sens.
a) embarcation b) ruminant vivant au Tibet
c) abominable homme des neiges   d) monnaie

11. Associez **paélia** et **goulache** à leur sens.
a) ragout de bœuf b) plat de riz, moules, poisson

12. Associez **calife** et **sanscrit** à leur sens.
a) chef musulman b) coupe sacrée c) langue sacrée

13. Associez **parafer** et **persiffler** à leur sens.
a) tuer b) ridiculiser c) apposer ses initiales d) crier

14. Associez **rapsodie** et **vilénie** à leur sens.
a) musique improvisée b) bassesse c) séjour (repos)

15. Associez **bélouga** et **bernard-l'ermite**.
a) crustacé b) pieuvre c) insecte d) baleine blanche

16. Associez **téléférique** et **téléférage**.
a) procédé de transport par câbles aériens
b) dispositif, moyen de transport par câbles aériens

17. Associez **asséner** et **réfréner** à leur sens.
a) nettoyer b) ralentir c) frapper brutalement

18. Associez **cleptomane** et **riquiqui**.
a) voleur   b) menteur   c) trop petit ou mesquin

Exercice récapitulatif 6

Je révise

RÈGLES A à G

Encerclez les formes recommandées et rayez les formes non recommandées.

(pagaille)
~~pagaye~~
~~pagaïe~~

althæa
althéa
altéa

béluga
bélouga
beluga

globetrotteur
globe-trotteur
globe-trotter

chiche-kébab
chichekébab
shishkebab

gilde
ghilde
guilde

hachich
haschich
haschisch

à capella
a capella
a cappella

et cætera
et cetera
etcétéra

goulash
goulache
goulasch

Toutes les formes ci-dessus existent. Avez-vous su lesquelles choisir? Réponses page 207.

trait d'union et soudure — singulier et pluriel — accents et tréma

par Chantal Contant

★ JEU — Dictée trouée

Demandez à l'un de vos proches d'aller au www.nouvelleorthographe.info/dictee.html et de vous dicter les mots à inscrire ci-dessous.

1. Je mange ce bon _p_____

avec une _c_____ .

2. Mon _p_____ émet

un _c_____ .

3. Ce _c_____

fait partie de la _m_____ locale.

4. J'ai cru _e_____

trois _c_____ sur la table.

5. C'est triste, car c'est fini. _S_____ !

Corrigez-vous. Puis, préparez-vous à l'examen final afin d'obtenir la meilleure note possible.

D'abord, révisez bien les règles et les mots, pour mettre toutes les chances de votre côté.

Voyez aussi la liste de 500 mots (p. 167-184). Elle vous aidera à visualiser les changements.

consonnes doubles   anomalies rectifiées   choix recommandés

Examen final
Mesurez vos progrès!

Je m'évalue

TOUTES LES RÈGLES

Maintenant que vous avez fait tous les tests et exercices de ce livre, revoyez bien les règles, puis faites cet examen final.

À quel pourcentage êtes-vous capable d'écrire selon l'orthographe moderne recommandée? À vous de voir…

Encerclez la forme recommandée.

▶ Selon les règles, il est préférable d'écrire…

1. a) **boursouffler**   b) **boursoufler**
2. a) **contre-filet**   b) **contrefilet**
3. a) **acuponcture**   b) **acupuncture**
4. a) **des matchs**   b) **des matches**
5. a) **grelotter**   b) **greloter**
6. a) **ultraviolet**   b) **ultra-violet**
7. a) **des caméras vidéo** b) **des caméras vidéos**
8. a) **événement**   b) **évènement**
9. a) **canette**   b) **cannette**

trait d'union et soudure | singulier et pluriel | accents et tréma

10. a) cardiovasculaire   b) cardio-vasculaire
11. a) il exagèrera   b) il exagérera
12. a) pique-niquer   b) piqueniquer
13. a) s'il vous plait   b) s'il vous plaît
14. a) un cure-dent   b) un cure-dents
15. a) interpeller   b) interpeler
16. a) base-ball   b) baseball
17. a) renouvellement   b) renouvèlement
18. a) vingt-et-un   b) vingt et un
19. a) assoir   b) asseoir
20. a) une note aiguë   b) une note aigüe
21. a) quincailler   b) quincaillier
22. a) shampooing   b) shampoing
23. a) j'époussette   b) j'époussète
24. a) pizzéria   b) pizzeria
25. a) il les a laissé rire   b) il les a laissés rire

Les réponses sont données en ligne sur le site www.nouvelleorthographe.info/corrige.html.

Ma note finale : _____ /25

Ma note en pourcentage (× 4) = _____ %

consonnes doubles   anomalies rectifiées   choix recommandés

500 mots courants

Voici 500 mots fréquents relevant des règles de l'orthographe recommandée. Pour illustrer une variété de cas différents, les mots d'une même famille n'ont pas tous été répertoriés.

Il faut comprendre que **boursouffler** englobe **boursoufflement** et **boursoufflure** ; que le verbe **apparaitre** inclut **apparait**, **apparaitra**, **apparaitrait** ; que **minijupe** dans la liste est un exemple pour **minichaine**, **minigolf**, etc.

Il existe des listes beaucoup plus complètes.

Pour consulter ces listes utiles lorsque vous rédigez ou que vous corrigez, procurez-vous l'un des ouvrages de référence présentés à la page 200 : ***La liste simplifiée*** (4 000 mots) ou alors le ***Grand vadémécum*** (beaucoup plus détaillé).

Liste de 500 mots courants

Afin d'énumérer le plus grand nombre possible d'exemples de mots fréquents, les mots de même famille et les mots similaires n'ont pas tous été listés ici. Ils suivent cependant la même règle. Ex. : **abat-vent** suit la même règle que **abat-jour**, **abime** perd son accent comme **abimer**, **accélèrerait** s'écrit comme **accélèrera**.

NON RECOMMANDÉ	RECOMMANDÉ	Page
	A	
abat-jour inv.	abat-jour(s)	56
abîmer	abimer	78
à cap(p)ella	à capella	88/141
accélérera	accélèrera	70
acupuncture	acuponcture	140
aérera	aèrera	70
affûter	affuter	78
aide-mémoire inv.	aide-mémoire(s)	56

NON RECOMMANDÉ	RECOMMANDÉ	Page
assidûment	assidument	78
asseoir	assoir	122
audio-visuel	audiovisuel	20
auto-analyse	autoanalyse	20
auto-école	autoécole	141
auto-évaluation	autoévaluation	20
avant-goût	avant-gout	78
avant-midi inv.	avant-midi(s)	56
→	→	

aigu, aiguë	aigu, aiguë		
aîné	aîné		
allègement	allègement	84	
allégement	allégement	78	
allo	allô	74	
ambigu, ambiguë	ambigu, ambiguë	74	
ambiguïté	ambiguïté	140	
anévrisme	anévrisme	84	
anti-douleur(s)	anti-douleur inv.	84	
anti-inflammatoire	anti-inflammatoire	141	
anti-oxydant	antioxydant	20/141	
anti-rides	anti-rides	20	
antiride(s)	antiride(s)	20	
août	août	20/141	
apparaître	apparaître	78	
appuie-tête(s)	appuie-tête inv.	78	
après-midi(s)	après-midi inv.	56	
assèchement	assèchement	56	
		74	

B		
balloter	ballotter	112
baseball	base-ball	24
basfond	bas-fond	28
basketball	basket-ball	24
bassecour(s)	basse(s)-cour(s)	28
béluga	béluga ou béluga	88/140
bienaimé	bien-aimé	28
bienêtre(s)	bien-être inv.	28
bienfondé	bien-fondé	28
bigbang(s)	big(-)bang inv.	24/62
bio(s)	bio adj. inv.	141
boite	boîte	78
boursoufler	boursoufler	122
boutentrain(s)	boute-en-train inv.	34/141
branlebas	branle-bas	34
brise-glace(s)	brise-glace inv.	56

500 mots courants

Le pluriel est indiqué entre parenthèses, et *inv.* signifie invariable.
Le numéro renvoie à la page où la règle est expliquée dans ce livre.

169

Orthographe recommandée : exercices et mots courants
par Chantal Contant

www.nouvelleorthographe.info
www.chantalcontant.info

NON RECOMMANDÉ	RECOMMANDÉ	Page
broncho-pneumonie	bronchopneumonie	20
brûlant	brulant	78
brûler	bruler	78
brûlure	brulure	78
bûche	buche	78
bûcher	bucher	78
bûcheron	bucheron	78

c

cacahuète	cacahouète	140
cache-cache inv.	cachecache(s)	24
cache-cou inv.	cache-cou(s)	56
cashmere	cachemire	141
cachotterie	cachoterie	112
cachottier	cachotier	112
cafeteria/cafétéria	cafétéria	88
↓		

NON RECOMMANDÉ	RECOMMANDÉ	Page
chauve(s)-souris	chauvesouris	34
chic adj. inv.	chic(s)	62
ci-gît	ci-git	78
ciné-parc	cinéparc	20
clef	clé	141
kleptomane	cleptomane	141
cliquettement	cliquètement	98
clopin-clopant	clopin-clopant	34
co-fondateur	cofondateur	20
coin-coin inv.	coincoin(s)	24
combatif	combattif	122
combativité	combattivité	122
comparaître	comparaitre	78
complètera	complétera	70
compte-gouttes	compte-goutte(s)	56
connaître	connaitre	78
↓		

170

cahin-caha	24	considérera	70
kaléidoscope	141	contre-attaque	12
khalife	141	contre-choc	12
ca͟nette	141	contre-cœur (à)	12
canoë	141	contre-jour	12
cañon	141	contremaître	78
cardio-vasculaire	20	contre-plaqué	12
casse-noisette(s)	56	contre-exemple	12
casse-tête(s)	56	contre-indication	12
cèdera	70	contre-interroger	12
cedex	141	contre-offensive	12
célébrera	70	corollaire	108
céleri	74	corolle	108
chaîne	78	couguar	
chariot	122	coupe-feu inv.	
chasse-neige(s)	56	coupe-ongles	
chauffe-eau(x)	56	coupe-vent inv.	

cahin-caha		considérera	
kaléidoscope		contrattaque	12
khalife		contrechoc	12
calife		contrecœur (à)	12
cannette		contrejour	12
canoé		contremaître	78
canyon		contreplaqué	12
cardiovasculaire		contrexemple	12
casse-noisette(s)		contrindication	12
casse-tête(s)		contrinterroger	12
cédera		controffensive	12
cédex		corolaire	108
célèbrera		corole	108
cèleri		cougar ou cougouar	140
chaine		coupe-feu(x)	56
charriot		coupe-ongle(s)	56
chasse-neige(s)		coupe-vent(s)	56
chauffe-eau(x)			

500 mots courants

Le pluriel est indiqué entre parenthèses, et *inv.* signifie invariable.
Le numéro renvoie à la page où la règle est expliquée dans ce livre.

Orthographe recommandée : exercices et mots courants
par Chantal Contant

NON RECOMMANDÉ	RECOMMANDÉ	Page
courbaturer	courbatturer	122
coût	cout	78
coûter	couter	78
coûteux	couteux	78
couvre-pieds	couvrepieds	34
couvre-sol inv.	couvre-sol(s)	56
cow-boy	cowboy	24
crèmerie	crémerie	74
crescendo inv.	crescendo(s)	62
croître, croîtra	croitre, croitra	78
croque-monsieur(s)	croquemonsieur(s)	34
croque-monsieur inv.	croquemonsieur inv.	34
croque-mort	croquemort	34
croûte	croute	78
croûton	crouton	78
crûment	crument	78
cuiller	cuillère	141

→

NON RECOMMANDÉ	RECOMMANDÉ	Page
dissous, dissoute	dissout, dissoute	122
don Juan (un)	donjuan (un)	24
dribbler	dribler	141
dûment	dument	78

E

NON RECOMMANDÉ	RECOMMANDÉ	Page
éco-centre	écocentre	20
ego inv.	égo(s)	62/88
électro-choc	électrochoc	20
emboîter	emboiter	78
embûche	embuche	78
emmenthal	emmental	140
enchaîner	enchainer	78
ensorcellement	ensorcèlement	98
ensorcelle (j')	ensorcèle (j')	98
en-tête (un)	entête (un)	34

→

172

cumulo-nimbus	cumulonimbus	20	
cure-dents	cure-dent(s)	56	
cyclo-tourisme	cyclotourisme	20	
D	**D**		
déboîter	déboiter	78	
décédera	décèdera	70	
déchaîner	déchainer	78	
dégoût	dégout	78	
dégoûtant	dégoutant	78	
dénivellement	dénivèlement	98	
dénivelle (je)	dénivèle (je)	98	
déplaît (il)	déplait (il)	78	
diesel	diésel	88	
digérera	digèrera	70	
dîner	diner	78	
disparaître	disparaitre	78	

entraîner	entrainer	20	entraîner	entrainer	78
entraîneur	entraineur	56	entraîneur	entraineur	78
entre-jambes	entrejambe(s)	20	entre-jambes	entrejambe(s)	12
entre-temps	entretemps		entre-temps	entretemps	12
entre-tuer (s')	entretuer (s')		entre-tuer (s')	entretuer (s')	12
entr'ouvrir	entrouvrir	78	entr'ouvrir	entrouvrir	12
envoûter	envouter	70	envoûter	envouter	78
époussette (j')	époussète (j')	78	époussette (j')	époussète (j')	98
espèrera	espérera	78	espèrera	espérera	70
essuie-glace inv.	essuie-glace(s)	78			
essuie-mains	essuie-main(s)	98			
essuie-tout inv.	essuietout(s)	98			
œstrogène	estrogène	78			
et cætera/et cetera	etcétéra(s) 24/62/88/140				
étincelle (j')	étincèle (j') verbe	88			
étiquette (j')	étiquète (j') verbe	70			
événement	évènement	78			

500 mots courants

Le pluriel est indiqué entre parenthèses, et *inv.* signifie invariable.
Le numéro renvoie à la page où la règle est expliquée dans ce livre.

173

Orthographe recommandée : exercices et mots courants
par Chantal Contant

NON RECOMMANDÉ	RECOMMANDÉ	Page
exagérera	exagèrera	70
eczéma	exéma	122
extra-fort	extrafort	16
extra-terrestre	extraterrestre	16
F		
fac-similé	facsimilé	24
faire-part inv.	fairepart(s)	34
feuillette (je)	feuillète (je)	98
fjord	fiord	141
flûte	flute	78
fourre-tout inv.	fourretout(s)	34
fox-trot inv.	foxtrot(s)	24/62
fraîche	fraiche	78
fraîcheur	fraicheur	78
frisotter	frisoter	112

NON RECOMMANDÉ	RECOMMANDÉ	Page
guru	gourou	140
goût	gout	78
goûter	gouter	78
graffiti inv.	graffiti(s)	62
granit	granite	141
gratte-ciel inv.	gratte-ciel(s)	56
grelottement	grelotement	112
grelotter	greloter	112
gri(s)-gri(s)	grigri(s)	24
grille-pain inv.	grille-pain(s)	56
grizzly/grizzlies	grizzli(s)	62/141
guérillero	guérilléro	88
H		
haschich/haschisch	hachich	141
hand-ball	handball	24

www.nouvelleorthographe.info
www.chantalcontant.info

frisottis	frisotti**s**	hara-kiri	ha<u>ra</u>kiri	24
frou(s)-frou(s)	froufrou(s)	haut(s)-fond(s)	hau<u>t</u>fond(s)	28
fût (ex. : bière en fut)	78	haut-parleur(s)	hau<u>t</u>parleur(s)	28
		hors-jeu inv.	hors-jeu(x)	56
G		hot(-)dog inv.	hotdog(s)	24/62
gageure	gageüre	84	hurrah !	hourra !	140
gaîté ou gaieté	gaité	78/141	huître	huitre	78
garde(s)-côte	garde-côte(s)	56	hydro-électricité	hydroélectricité	20
garde(s)-malade(s)	garde-malade(s)	56			
garde(s)-pêche	garde-pêche(s)	56	**I**		
garde-manger inv.	garde-manger(s)	56	igloo	iglou	140
gastro-entérite	gastroentérite	20	île	ile	78
gelinotte	gélinotte	130	îlot	ilot	78
gérera	gèrera	70	imbécillité	imbécilité	122
giga-octet	gigaoctet	20	impresario/impresarii	imprésario(s)	62/88
gîte	gite	78	hindou, hindoue	<u>h</u>indou, <u>h</u>indoue	140
globe-trotter	globetrotteur	24/141	indûment	ind<u>u</u>ment	78

500 mots courants

Le pluriel est indiqué entre parenthèses, et *inv* signifie invariable.
Le numéro renvoie à la page où la règle est expliquée dans ce livre.

175

Orthographe recommandée : exercices et mots courants
par Chantal Contant

NON RECOMMANDÉ	RECOMMANDÉ	Page
in extremis	in extrêmis	88
infra-rouge	infrarouge	16
inquiètera	inquièterra	70
insèrera	insèrera	70
intègrera	intègrera	70
interpeller	interpeler	104
interviewer n.m.	intervieweur	141
intra-artériel	intraartériel	16
intra-veineuse	intraveineuse	16

J

jeans (un/des)	jean (un), des jeans	62
jeûner, jeûnons	jeuner, jeunons	78
	mais jeûne, jeûnes	78
joaillier, joaillière	joailler, joaillère	130
jumelle (je)	jumèle (je) verbe	98

NON RECOMMANDÉ	RECOMMANDÉ	Page
maffia	mafia	141
maffioso/maffiosi	mafioso(s)	62/141
mahara(dja(h)	maharadja	140/141
main-forte (prêter)	mainforte (prêter)	34
maître	maitre	78
maîtresse	maitresse	78
maîtriser	maitriser	78
mal famé	malfamé	28
mange-tout inv.	mangetout(s)	34
maniaco-dépressif	maniacodépressif	20
marguillier	marguiller	130
match(es)	match(s)	62
maximum/maxima	maximum(s)	62
médico-légal	médicolégal	20
méga-octet	mégaoctet	20
méli(s)-mélo(s)	mélimélo(s)	24

kilo-octet		micro-économie	20
kilooctet	20	micro-ondes (four)	141
kirsch	141	micro-organisme	20
lance-flammes		mille-feuille	28
lance-flamme(s)	56	mille-pattes	28
lance-missiles		mini-jupe	20
lance-missile(s)	56	minimum/minima	62
land/des länder		modèrera	70
land(s)	62	monorail inv.	
lave-vaisselle inv.		moto-neige	70
lave-vaisselle(s)	56	mouffette	141
léchera	70	multi-ethnique	20
levrault		multi-sports adj.	
levreau	122	multi-sport(s) adj.	20/141
libèrera	70	mûr, mûre adj.,	
lis	141	mûrs, mûres	
ludo-éducatif		mûre n.f. (le fruit)	
ludoéducatif	20	mûrir	
lunch(es)			
lunch(s)	62		
M			
macaroni inv.			
macaroni(s)	62		
macro-économie			
macroéconomie	20		

		microéconomie	20
		microonde(s)	20/141
		microorganisme	20
		millefeuille	28
		millepatte(s)	28
		minijupe	20
		minimum(s)	62
		modèrera	70
		monorail(s)	141
		motoneige	20
		moufette	141
		multiethnique	20
		multisport(s)	20/141
		mûr, mûre adj.,	
		mûrs, mûres	
		mure n.f. (le fruit)	78
		murir	78

---

500 mots courants

Le pluriel est indiqué entre parenthèses, et *inv.* signifie invariable.
Le numéro renvoie à la page où la règle est expliquée dans ce livre.

177

Orthographe recommandée : exercices et mots courants
par Chantal Contant

www.nouvelleorthographe.info
www.chantalcontant.info

178

NON RECOMMANDÉ	RECOMMANDÉ	Page
	N	
naître	naitre	78
néanderthalien	néandertalien	140
nénuphar	nénufar	122
néo-brunswickois	néobrunswickois	20
néo-démocrate	néodémocrate	20
néo-libéralisme	néolibéralisme	20
néo-zélandais	néozélandais	20
nippon, nipponne	nippon, nippone	141
nirvâna	nirvana	140
nivèlement	nivèlement	98
nivelle (je)	nivèle (je) verbe	98
	O	
oignon	ognon	122
omni-sports adj.	omnisport(s)	20/141
→		

NON RECOMMANDÉ	RECOMMANDÉ	Page
pare-soleil inv.	pare-soleil(s)	56
passe-boules	passe-boule(s)	56
passe-partout inv.	passepartout(s)	35
passe-temps	passetemps	42
pêcheresse	pêcheresse	74
pee(-)wee inv.	peewee(s)	24/62
pêle-mêle inv.	pêlemêle(s)	24
pénétrera	pénètrera	70
pepperoni	pepéroni	88
perce-neige inv.	perce-neige(s)	56
persiffler	persifler	122
pèse-personne inv.	pèse-personne(s)	56
phœnix (palmier)	phénix	140
pique-nique	piquenique	34
pique-niquer	piqueniquer	34
piqûre	piqure	78
→		

opèrera	opèrera	pizzeria	pizzéria	88
oto-rhino-laryngologiste	otorhinolaryngologiste	plaît (il)	plaît (il)	78
ouvre-boîtes	ouvre-boîte(s)	56/78	plate(s)-bande(s)	platebande(s)	141
ouvre-bouteilles	ouvre-bouteille(s)	56	plate(s)-forme(s)	plateforme(s)	141
		pluri-ethnique	pluriethnique	20
		porte-avions	porte-avion(s)	56
P		porte-bonheur inv.	porte-bonheur(s)	56
paella ou paëlla	paélia	141	porte-clés / -clefs	porteclé(s)	42/141
panini inv.	panini(s)	62	porte-manteau	portemanteau	42
paparazzi inv.	paparazzi(s)	62	porte-monnaie inv.	portemonnaie(s)	42
paraître	paraitre	78	porte-parole inv.	porte-parole(s)	56
para-médical	paramédical	20	porte-voix	portevoix	42
para-scolaire	parascolaire	20	possèdera	possèdera	70
pare-balles	pare-balle(s)	56	post-moderne	postmoderne	20
pare-brise inv.	parebrise(s)	42	post-production	postproduction	20
pare-chocs	parechoc(s)	42	pot(s)-pourri(s)	potpourri(s)	34
pare-étincelles	pare-étincelle(s)	56	pudding	pouding	140/141

500 mots courants Le pluriel est indiqué entre parenthèses, et *inv.* signifie invariable.
Le numéro renvoie à la page où la règle est expliquée dans ce livre.

179

Orthographe recommandée : exercices et mots courants
par Chantal Contant

www.nouvelleorthographe.info
www.chantalcontant.info

180

NON RECOMMANDÉ	RECOMMANDÉ	Page
pré-adolescence	préadolescence	20
pré-autorisation	préautorisation	20
précèdera	précédera	70
pré-électoral	préélectoral	20
pré-emballé	préemballé	20
préfèrera	préférera	70
pré-maternelle	prématernelle	20
presqu'île	presqu'ile	78
presse-ail inv.	presse-ail(s)	56
presse-citron inv.	presse-citron(s)	56
presse-fruits	presse-fruit(s)	56
pré-traitement	prétraitement	20
pré-universitaire	préuniversitaire	20
prima donna inv.	primadonna(s)	24/62
pro-actif	proactif	20
procèdera	procédera	70

→

NON RECOMMANDÉ	RECOMMANDÉ	Page
rafraîchir	rafraichir	78
rafraîchissant	rafraichissant	78
ragoût	ragout	78
rasseoir	rassoir	122
ravioli inv.	ravioli(s)	62
réapparaître	réapparaitre	78
reconnaître	reconnaitre	78
récupèrera	récupérera	70
referendum	référendum	88
réfètera	réfétera	70
reflètera	reflétera	70
règlementation	réglementation	74
règlementer	réglementer	74
règlera	réglera	70
règnera	régnera	70
relais	relai	122

→

prospérera	70	prospèrera	
protège-cou inv.	56	protège-cou(s)	
protège-genou	56	protège-genou(x)	
protégera	70	protègera	
pseudo-science	20	pseudoscience	
psycho-affectif	20	psychoaffectif	
psycho-éducation	20	psychoéducation	

Q

québécois	130	québécois	
quincaillier	130	quincailler	

R

rabat-joie inv.	56	rabat-joie(s)	56
radio-actif	20	radioactif	20
radio-journal	20	radiojournal	20
radio-oncologie	20	radiooncologie	20

remue-ménage inv.	remue-ménage(s)	56
renaître	renaître	78
renouvellement	renouvèlement	98
renouvelle (je)	renouvèle (je)	98
répétera	répètera	70
repose-pieds	repose-pied(s)	56
résonnant adj.	résonant	141
rétro-action	rétroaction	20
rétro-projecteur	rétroprojecteur	20
réveille-matin inv.	réveille-matin(s)	56
révélera	révèlera	70
revolver	révolver	88
rince-bouche inv.	rince-bouche(s)	56
rond(s)-point(s)	rondpoint(s)	34
rouspétera	rouspètera	70
ruissellement	ruissèlement	98
ruisselle (je)	ruissèle (je)	98

500 mots courants

Le pluriel est indiqué entre parenthèses, et *inv.* signifie invariable.
Le numéro renvoie à la page où la règle est expliquée dans ce livre.

181

Orthographe recommandée : exercices et mots courants
par Chantal Contant

www.nouvelleorthographe.info
www.chantalcontant.info

182

NON RECOMMANDÉ	RECOMMANDÉ	Page
S	**S**	
sac_charine	sac_carine	122
sacro-saint	sacrosaint	20
sage(s)-femme(s)	sagefemme(s)	34
sandwich(es)	sandwich(s)	62
sans-abri inv.	sans-abri(s)	56
sans-cœur inv.	sans-cœur(s)	56
sans-papiers	sans-papier(s)	56
sauf-conduit	saufconduit	34
scenario/scenarii	scénario(s)	62/88
sèchera	séchera	70
sècheresse	sécheresse	74
senior	sénior	88
sequoia	séquoia	88
serpillière	serpillière	130
servo-frein	servofrein	20
→		

NON RECOMMANDÉ	RECOMMANDÉ	Page
stimulus/stimuli	stimulus (un/des)	62
succédera	succèdera	70
suggérera	suggèrera	70
super-production	superproduction	20
sûr, sûre (certaine),	sûr, sûre (certaine),	78
sûrs, sûres	sûrs, sûres	78
sûrement	sûrement	78
sûreté	sûreté	78
T	**T**	
taï-chi ou taï-chi	taïchi	24/141
taille-crayon inv.	taille-crayon(s)	56
tam-tam inv.	tamtam(s)	24
tannin	tanin	141
ciao !	tchao !	141
tchin-tchin !	tchintchin !	24
	→	

shampooing	141	shampoing	141
siégera	70	siègera	20
s'il te plaît	78	s'il te plait	20
s'il vous plaît	78	s'il vous plait	20
socio-culturel	20	socioculturel	20
socio-économique	20	socioéconomique	20
sombréro	88	sombrero	88
soprano/soprani	62	soprano(s)	62
souffre-douleur inv.	56	souffre-douleur(s)	34
soûl ou saoul	78/141	soul	24
soûler ou saouler	78/141	souler	42
sous-verre inv.	56	sous-verre(s)	42
spaghetti inv.	62	spaghetti(s)	56
spatio-temporel	20	spatiotemporel	70
sprinter n.m.	141	sprintera	56
standard adj. inv.	62	standard(s)	78
statu quo inv.	24/62	statuquo(s)	78

téléphérique		téléférique	141
télé-film		téléfilm	20
télé-journal		téléjournal	20
télé-objectif		téléobjectif	20
télé-réalité		téléréalité	20
tequila		téquila	88
terre-plein		terreplein	34
thaï(s)		thaï(s), thaïe(s)	62/141
tic(-)tac inv.		tictac(s)	24
tire-bouchon		tirebouchon	42
tire-bouchonner		tirebouchonner	42
tire-fesses		tire-fesse(s)	56
tolèrera		tolérera	70
tourne-disques		tourne-disque(s)	56
traîneau		traineau	78
traîne		traine	78
traître, traîtresse		traitre, traitresse	78

---

500 mots courants

Le pluriel est indiqué entre parenthèses, et *inv.* signifie invariable.
Le numéro renvoie à la page où la règle est expliquée dans ce livre.

183

Orthographe recommandée : exercices et mots courants
par Chantal Contant

www.nouvelleorthographe.info
www.chantalcontant.info

NON RECOMMANDÉ	RECOMMANDÉ	Page	NON RECOMMANDÉ	RECOMMANDÉ	Page
transférera	transfèrera	70	véto (droit de)	véto (droit de)	88
transparaître	transparaitre	78	vidéo adj. inv.	vidéo(s)	141
trimballer	trimbaler	141	vidéo-cassette	vidéocassette	20
trouble-fête inv.	trouble-fête(s)	56	vidéo-clip	vidéoclip	20
tue-mouche inv.	tue-mouche(s)	56	vidéo-conférence	vidéoconférence	20
			volley-ball	volleyball	24
			volte-face (faire)	volteface (faire)	34
	U		voûte	voute	78
ultra-son	ultrason	16			
ultra-violet	ultraviolet	16		**W-X**	
hululer	ululer	140	water-polo	waterpolo	24
			week-end	weekend	24
	V				
vade-mecum inv.	vadémécum(s)	24/62/88		**Y-Z**	
va-nu-pieds	vanupied(s)	34	yoghourt ou yaourt	yogourt ou yaourt	140
varia inv.	varia(s)	62	youppi! ou youpie!	youpi!	141
végétera	végètera	70	yukonnais	yukonais	141
vélo-camping	vélocamping	141			

184

Les dictionnaires se mettent à jour

Aujourd'hui, beaucoup de dictionnaires récents ainsi que tous les grands correcteurs informatiques (Word, OpenOffice.org, Antidote, ProLexis...) reconnaissent ces graphies.

Vous pouvez consulter une liste de dictionnaires à jour au www.nouvelleorthographe.info.

Voici 15 exemples de mots dont l'orthographe a évolué (p. 186). La forme moderne de ces mots apparait dans la plupart des dictionnaires récents. Elle est donc reconnue.

Sur un échantillon de 10 dictionnaires, le tableau qui suit vous indique le nombre de fois que la graphie moderne est présente. Les 10 dictionnaires consultés* sont les suivants :

— *Petit Larousse*
— *Petit Robert*

— *Dictionnaire de l'Académie française*
— *Dictionnaire Hachette*
— *Dictionnaire du correcteur de Word*

— *Larousse des noms communs*
— *Dictionnaire d'orthographe et de difficultés du français* (éd. Le Robert)
— *Nouveau Petit Littré*
— *Dictionnaire Hachette Junior*
— *Dictionnaire électronique Antidote*

---

*Vous trouverez dans la bibliographie (pages 212-213) l'année d'édition de chaque dictionnaire consulté.

15 exemples dans 10 dictionnaires

Règle	Graphie traditionnelle non recommandée	Graphie moderne recommandée	Présence dans les **10** dictionnaires
1- soudure préfixe savant (p. 20)	cardio-vasculaire	cardiovasculaire*	9/10
2- soudure mot étranger (p. 24)	base-ball	baseball*	9/10
3- soudure avec mille- (p. 28)	un mille-pattes	un millepatte*	9/10
4- singulier régulier nom composé (p. 56)	un presse-papiers	un presse-papier*	9/10
5- pluriel régulier nom composé (p. 56)	des abat-jour	des abat-jours*	9/10
6- pluriel régulier mot étranger (p. 62)	des novæ ou des supernovæ	des novas* ou des supernovas*	9/10
7- accent grave (p. 74)	événement	évènement*	10/10

8- accent circonflexe sur **i** ou **u** (p. 78)	brûler	**bruler***	8/10
9- tréma déplacé sur le **u** (p. 84)	une voix aiguë	**une voix aigüe***	8/10
10- accent français mot étranger (p. 88)	pizzeria	**pizzéria***	9/10
11- consonne simple après **e** (p. 104)	interpeller	**interpeler***	9/10
12- famille harmonisée (p. 124)	combatif	**combattif***	9/10
13- série harmonisée (p. 125)	asseoir	**assoir***	8/10
14- anomalie rectifiée (p. 126)	douceâtre	**douçâtre***	9/10
15- finale -illier rectifiée en **-iller** (p. 130)	quincaillier ou joaillier	**quincailler*** ou **joailler***	9/10

* Les mots ont évolué et leurs nouvelles formes, plus régulières, sont désormais admises. Les graphies modernes ci-dessus étaient toutes absentes du *Petit Larousse Illustré* 1988 et du *Petit Robert 1* de 1990. Comme le montre ce tableau, presque tous les dictionnaires consultés les reconnaissent aujourd'hui ; vous pouvez donc les employer sans hésitation.

Précisions linguistiques

demi-, mi-, semi-, quasi(-)

Les préfixes **demi-**, **mi-**, **semi-**, **quasi**(-) ne sont pas touchés par les rectifications. On ne les soude jamais. On continue donc d'écrire :
- **une demi-heure** ;
- **la mi-décembre** ;
- **les cheveux mi-longs** ;
- **des semi-remorques** ;
- **une arme semi-automatique** ;
- **la quasi-certitude** (trait d'union devant le nom) ;
- **il est quasi certain** (espace devant l'adjectif).

Assurez-vous de porter une attention aux différences d'orthographe dans :
- **les yeux mi-ouverts** ;
- **les yeux à demi ouverts** (cas de : à demi) ;
- **deux heures et demie** (après le nom) ;

bien que ces subtilités ne relèvent pas des nouvelles règles.

En nouvelle orthographe, rappelez-vous qu'on soude **anti-**, **archi-**, **mini-** et aussi **maxi-** : **antiride, antiinflammatoire, antivirus, archiimportant, archiprudent, minichaine, minigolf, maxijupe**...

vice-, ex-, sous-, non(-)

Les éléments **vice-**, **ex-**, **sous-** et **non**(-) ne sont pas touchés. On continue donc d'écrire :
— le **vice-président** est son **ex-mari** ;
— ce **sous-produit** est **sous-utilisé** ;
— la **non-violence** (trait d'union devant le nom) ;
— il est **non violent** (espace devant l'adjectif).

Notez que **sous-tasse** pouvait déjà s'écrire **soutasse**, comme **soucoupe**. On choisit donc la forme en un mot (règle G19). Par contre, **sous-verre** ne connait qu'une seule façon de s'écrire. Rappelez-vous que **sur-** (**surutilisé**), **pré-**, **post-** et **télé-** sont soudés.

vingt et cent

La règle d'accord de **vingt** et **cent** n'est pas changée. On les accorde s'ils sont multipliés et qu'ils terminent le nombre :
— **deux-cents**, mais **deux-cent-quinze** ;
— **quatre-vingts**, mais **quatre-vingt-six**.

Noms propres

En principe, les noms propres (et les marques de commerce) ne sont pas touchés par les rectifications : **Nîmes**, **Sept-Îles**.

Démêlez le vrai du faux

Oui, la nouvelle orthographe...

☑ élimine des exceptions non justifiées.

☑ améliore la cohérence dans l'écriture.

☑ apporte régularisation et francisation.

☑ est de plus en plus dans les dictionnaires.

☑ est recommandée, sans être obligatoire.

Non, la nouvelle orthographe...

⊗ n'est pas une écriture phonétique.

⊗ ne cherche pas à niveler par le bas : elle renforce le système des règles du français.

⊗ n'a pas l'ampleur d'une « réforme » : ce sont de petits ajustements bien ciblés.

⊗ ne touche pas à la langue elle-même, mais à son système de transcription à l'écrit.

⊗ n'a pas eu pour but de résoudre les échecs scolaires, mais bien d'éliminer des anomalies.

Oui, on peut mélanger les deux

Les deux orthographes coexistent et sont admises. **On peut donc mélanger les deux orthographes dans un même texte** : c'est ce que font tous les gens qui écrivent, y compris vous-même, comme vous avez pu le constater dans les tests intuitifs.

À l'école, aucun élève ne peut être pénalisé pour avoir utilisé les graphies rectifiées, ni pour avoir mélangé l'orthographe traditionnelle et moderne dans un texte ou un examen, et ce, même pour un même mot.

Non, n'hésitez plus

N'hésitez plus à écrire en orthographe rectifiée dans vos textes personnels et au travail.

Étant donné que tous les grands correcteurs informatiques et beaucoup de dictionnaires sont à jour, pourquoi attendre?

Pour faire connaitre* votre décision, ajoutez au besoin une note en bas de page comme ici. Si l'un de vos lecteurs croit que vous avez commis une erreur, cette note servira à bien l'informer. Elle rassurera tout le monde.

---

*J'applique les changements apportés à l'orthographe. Ex. : *connaitre* sans accent (www.nouvelleorthographe.info).

Informations pratiques

Réglez votre correcteur

L'ajustement des **réglages** de votre logiciel de correction vous aidera grandement à être moderne.

Il vous **signalera** tout de suite les graphies non recommandées. Prenez le temps d'ajuster vos réglages (voir www.nouvelleorthographe.info).

Livres et sites

La page 212 (bibliographie) vous conseille des lectures à faire ou des sites à consulter. Les pages 193 et plus illustrent des livres utiles.

Informations gratuites

Vous pouvez recevoir gratuitement de l'information sur l'orthographe. Il suffit d'en faire la demande par messagerie électronique. Voyez www.nouvelleorthographe.info.

Vous pourrez aussi demander la **trousse gratuite d'autoformation (avec vidéos)** pour une formation sans frais en entreprise, dans un organisme ou à l'école.

Connaitre et maitriser la nouvelle orthographe
Guide pratique avec exercices

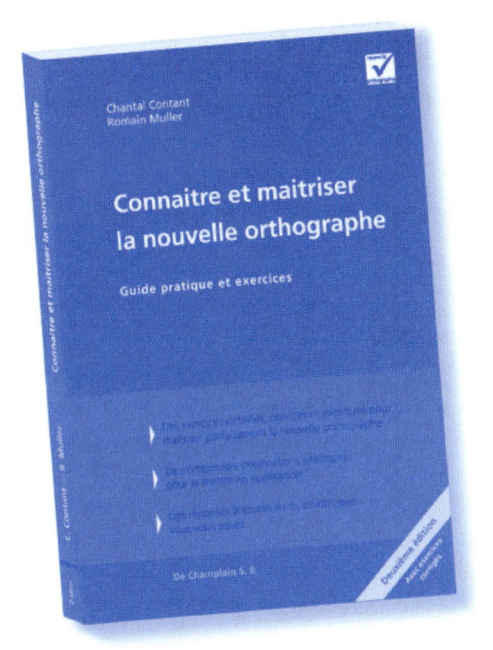

Le guide complet pour les enseignants et les professionnels de l'écriture

Des conseils utiles, des exercices approfondis avec justifications et tour d'horizon par règle, des interrogations et curiosités linguistiques.

Guide simplifié en couleurs

Les rectifications de l'orthographe du français

Simple, coloré et agréable à lire
(images intérieures illustrées à droite)

Ce livre en couleurs contient :

- des tableaux qui comparent l'ancienne et la nouvelle orthographe ;
- les règles et leur résumé ;
- plusieurs conseils pratiques pour la mise en application dans les écrits, au quotidien ;
- des bulles explicatives colorées attrayantes.

Un livre idéal pour le **grand public**, en **langage simple et clair** pour les employés de bureau, les parents, les élèves ou les personnes qui ne sont pas spécialistes de la langue française.

Des tableaux simples et en couleurs, des exemples qui se concentrent sur les mots courants, des encadrés attrayants. Bref, un livre facile d'accès, une initiation en douceur pour tout le monde !

Publié par De Boeck en Europe et par ERPI au Canada. Détails au www.chantalcontant.info.

Les rectifications de l'orthographe du français

La nouvelle orthographe accessible

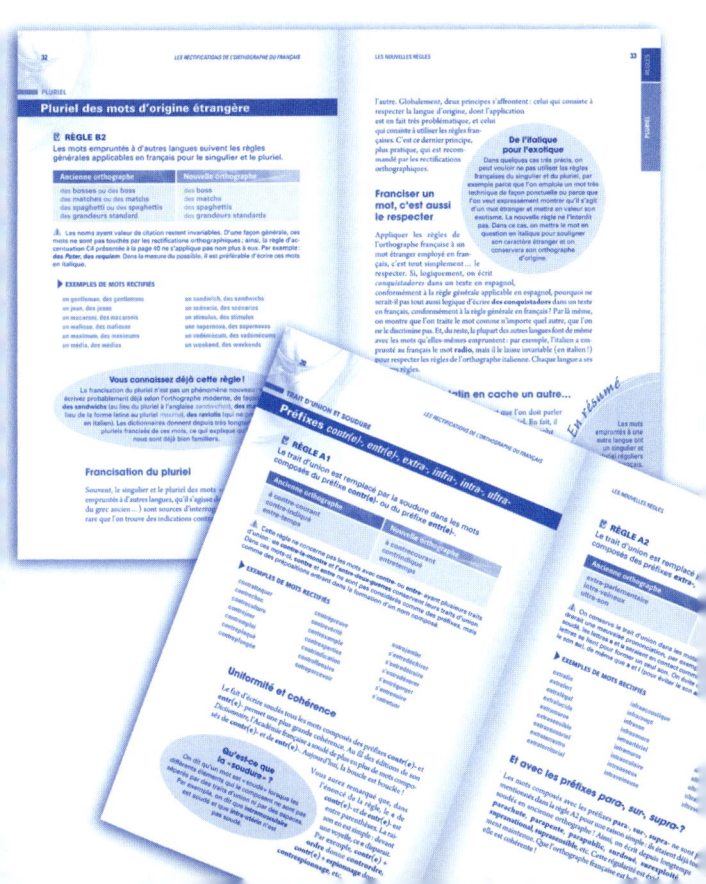

Le Verbe visite les pronoms
au village de La Phrase
conte éducatif

Suivez le roi *Le Verbe*
sur la rue Du Singulier
et la rue Du Pluriel pour
visiter les six boutiques
des pronoms.

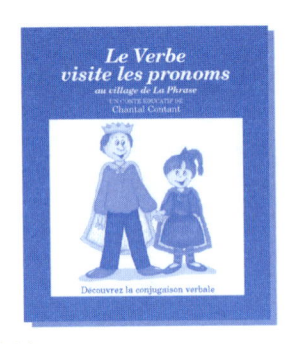

**Une conjugaison parfaite de plaisirs,
à partir de sept ans.**

Un apprentissage en douceur des terminaisons verbales.

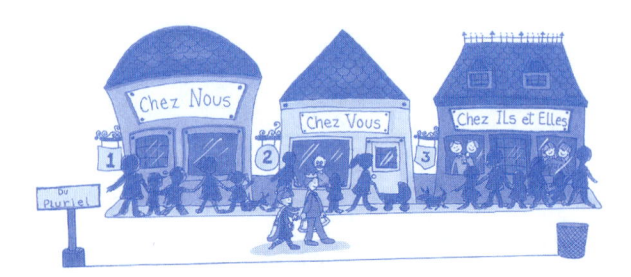

L'histoire amusante de Participe Passé
conte éducatif

Participe Passé adore être avec *Être*, son meilleur ami.
Il y a un parfait accord quand ils sont ensemble.

Le voisin *Avoir* est cependant beaucoup moins aimable.
Heureusement que marraine *Complément Direct* est là
pour faire régner l'accord.

L'enfant apprendra à son insu les règles de base de
l'accord du participe passé en français lorsqu'il fera
connaissance avec les personnages de ce conte éducatif.

**Une façon simple
d'apprendre les règles
du participe passé
et de mettre fin
aux problèmes d'accord.**

Pour tous les âges.

En librairie en Europe
et au Canada.

www.dechamplain.ca/livres

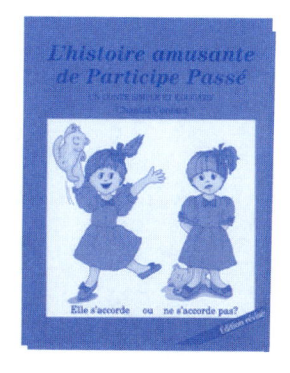

Les habitants du village de La Phrase
conte éducatif

Une initiation aux classes de mots.

Pour les enfants de six ans et plus.

Dans ce conte, le roi *Le Verbe* cherche un sujet.
En parcourant le pays du Texte, il rencontrera toutes les classes de mots.

L'enfant fera connaissance avec le *Nom Commun*, son meilleur ami le chien *Déterminant*, ses copains les *Adjectifs*, les fous du roi appelés les *Adverbes*, etc.

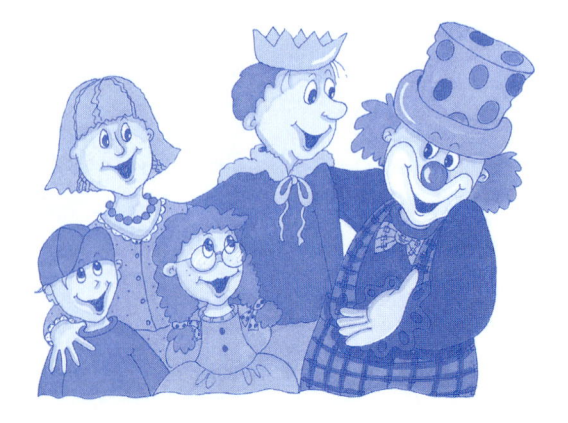

Contes éducatifs amusants

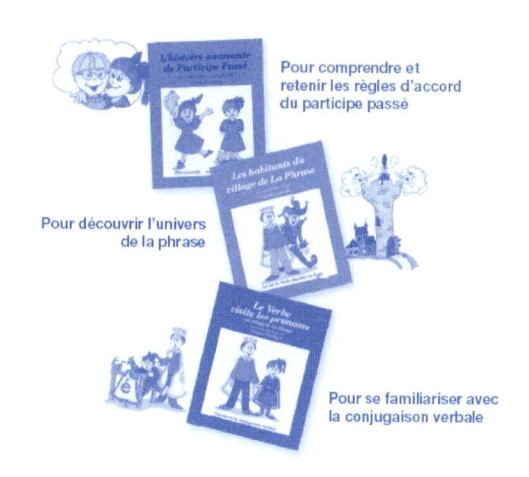

Pour comprendre et retenir les règles d'accord du participe passé

Pour découvrir l'univers de la phrase

Pour se familiariser avec la conjugaison verbale

→ **Tous les détails au www.chantalcontant.info.**

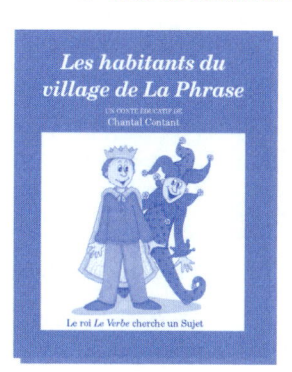

√ **Une trousse pédagogique** permet de guider judicieusement les enseignants qui utilisent ce conte en classe pour familiariser leurs élèves avec les différentes catégories de mots dans la phrase. Pour se procurer la trousse, voir www.dechamplain.ca/livres.

√ Ce conte éducatif existe aussi en **version cédérom** pour l'école ou la maison.

La référence en orthographe

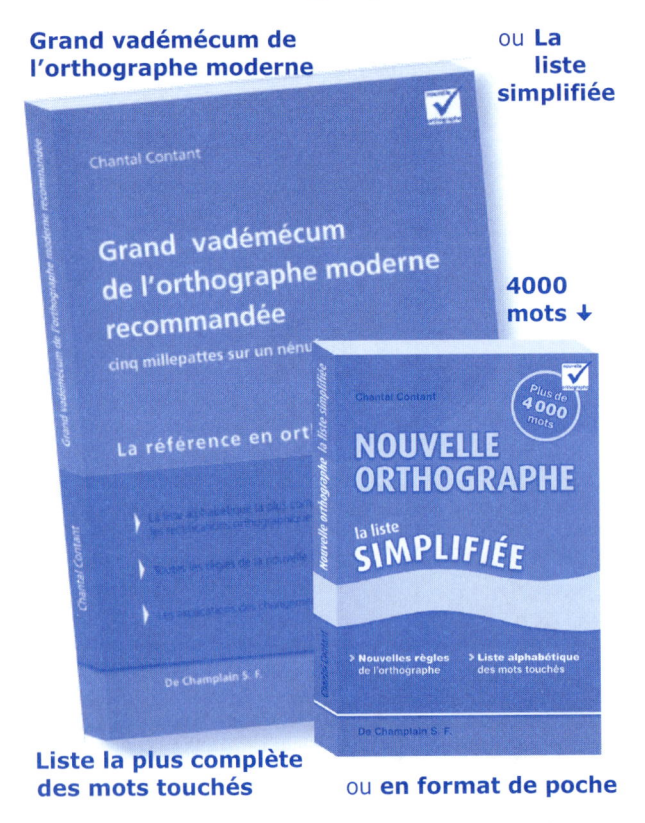

Grand vadémécum de l'orthographe moderne

ou **La liste simplifiée**

4000 mots ↓

Liste la plus complète des mots touchés

ou **en format de poche**

Pour rédiger, corriger, réviser, enseigner, traduire, afin de vérifier tous les mots rectifiés (en librairie).

Corrigé des tests intuitifs

Vous trouverez dans les pages 202 à 205 les réponses recommandées pour tous les tests intuitifs « **Je me teste** ». À l'étape 4 de chaque test, vous aurez ces réponses écrites au long.

Interprétation des résultats

CALCULEZ VOTRE RÉSULTAT
Comparez vos réponses à celles des pages suivantes et notez-y votre résultat.

FORMES RECOMMANDÉES
Plus votre résultat se rapproche de 10 dans un test intuitif, plus vous appliquez spontanément les principes de la règle dans vos écrits. Vous écrivez déjà de façon moderne.

FORMES TRADITIONNELLES (NON RECOMMANDÉES)
Si vous n'avez pas eu 10/10, vous n'avez pas nécessairement commis des erreurs d'orthographe. Certaines formes dites traditionnelles sont encore admises, et il est probable que vous employiez encore certaines d'entre elles.

FORMES FAUTIVES EN FRANÇAIS
Dans les tests, certaines formes sont fautives (donc incorrectes en français, inexistantes, interdites). On vous demandera à l'étape 4 de chaque règle d'aller les rayer : vous ne devez jamais les employer.

◆ Règle A1 (p. 11)   Ma note :   /10
Soudure : **contr(e)-** et **entr(e)-**

1b, 2b, 3b, 4b, 5a, 6b, 7b, 8b, 9b, 10b

◆ Règle A2 (p. 15)   Ma note :   /10
Soudure : **extra-, infra-, intra-** et **ultra-**

1b, 2b, 3a, 4b, 5b, 6b, 7a, 8b, 9b, 10b

◆ Règle A3 (p. 19)   Ma note :   /10
Soudure: éléments savants

1b, 2b, 3a, 4b, 5b, 6a, 7b, 8b, 9b, 10b

◆ Règle A4 (p. 23)   Ma note :   /10
Soudure : onomatopées et mots empruntés

1b, 2b, 3b, 4b, 5b, 6b, 7b, 8b, 9b, 10b

◆ Règle A5, 1re partie (p. 27)   Ma note :   /10
Bas(se)-, bien-, haut(e)-, mal- et **mille-**

1b, 2a, 3b, 4b, 5b, 6a, 7b, 8b, 9b, 10b

◆ Règle A5, 2e partie (p. 33)   Ma note :   /10
Soudure : **-tout** et autres soudures ciblées

1b, 2b, 3b, 4b, 5b, 6b, 7b, 8b, 9a, 10b

◆ Règle A5, 3e partie (p. 41)   Ma note :   /10
Soudure : **pare-, passe-, porte-** et **tire-**

1b, 2a, 3b, 4b, 5a, 6b, 7b, 8b, 9a, 10b

www.**nouvelle**orthographe.info

◆ **Règle A6** (p. 47)   Ma note :   /10
Traits d'union dans un numéral composé
1b, 2b, 3b, 4b, 5b, 6b, 7b, 8b, 9b, 10b

◆ **Règle B1** (p. 55)   Ma note :   /10
Singulier et pluriel des noms composés
1a, 2a, 3a, 4a, 5b, 6b, 7b, 8b, 9b, 10b

◆ **Règle B2** (p. 61)   Ma note :   /10
Singulier et pluriel des mots empruntés
1b, 2b, 3b, 4b, 5b, 6a, 7b, 8b, 9b, 10b

◆ **Règle C1**, 1re partie (p. 69) Ma note :   /10
Accent grave devant e : **cè**de**ra, cè**de**rait**...
1a, 2b, 3b, 4b, 5a, 6a, 7a, 8b, 9b, 10b

◆ **Règle C1**, 2e partie (p. 73) Ma note :   /10
Accent : orthographe **è** (et non **é**) devant **e**
1b, 2b, 3b, 4b, 5a, 6b, 7b, 8a, 9b, 10b

◆ **Règle C2** (p. 77)   Ma note :   /10
Accent circonflexe : disparition sur **i** et **u**
1b, 2b, 3a, 4b, 5b, 6a, 7b, 8a, 9b, 10a

◆ **Règle C3** (p. 83)   Ma note :   /10
Tréma déplacé ou ajouté dans quelques mots
1a, 2b, 3b, 4b, 5b, 6b, 7b, 8b, 9b, 10b

◆ Règle C4 (p. 87)   Ma note :   /10
Accents : mots empruntés francisés

1b, 2b, 3b, 4b, 5a, 6b, 7b, 8b, 9b, 10b

◆ Règle D1 (p. 97)   Ma note :   /10
-èle/-ète et **-èlement/-ètement**

1a, 2b, 3b, 4b, 5b, 6b, 7b, 8b, 9a, 10b

◆ Règle D2 (p. 103)   Ma note :   /10
Consonne simple après le son « e »

1a, 2a, 3b, 4b, 5b, 6b, 7a, 8b, 9a **ou** 9b, 10a **ou** 10b

◆ Règle D3, 1ʳᵉ partie (p. 107)   Ma note :   /10
Mots en **-ole** (et leur famille)

1b, 2b, 3b, 4b, 5b, 6b, 7b, 8b, 9b, 10a

◆ Règle D3, 2ᵉ partie (p. 111)   Ma note :   /10
Verbes en **-oter** (et leur famille)

1b, 2b, 3b, 4b, 5b, 6b, 7b, 8a, 9b, 10b

◆ Règles E, F1, F2 (p. 121)   Ma note :   /10
Participe passé **laissé**, et anomalies rectifiées pour harmoniser des familles ou des séries

1a, 2a, 3b, 4b, 5a, 6b, 7a, 8a, 9b, 10a

◆ Règles F3 et F4 (p. 129)   Ma note :   /10
Accents manquants et mots en **-iller/-illère**

1b, 2b, 3b, 4b, 5a **ou** 5b, 6a **ou** 6b, 7b, 8b, 9b, 10b

♦ **Règles G** (p. 139)   Ma note : /10
Forme recommandée à choisir entre deux formes déjà existantes

1a, 2b, 3a, 4a, 5b, 6b, 7a, 8a, 9b, 10a

♦ ♦ ♦ ♦ ♦

Quelles sont les règles que vous appliquez le <u>mieux</u> spontanément dans vos écrits ?

Ce sont les règles pour lesquelles votre résultat au test intuitif se rapproche le plus de 10/10.

Bravo à vous pour ces règles ! Vous employez **déjà** les formes qui sont recommandées.

Quelles sont les règles que vous appliquez le <u>moins</u> spontanément dans vos écrits ?

Ce sont les règles pour lesquelles votre résultat au test intuitif est de 5/10 ou moins.

Revoyez bien ces règles si vous souhaitez écrire davantage selon l'orthographe moderne recommandée.

Corrigé des exercices récapitulatifs

Voici les formes recommandées qu'il fallait encercler dans les exercices récapitulatifs intitulés « **Je révise** ».

♦ Exercice récapitulatif 1 (p. 67)

Règles A et B
des croquemonsieurs
des graffitis
jeu de cachecache
des sans-gênes
à contrecourant
un weekend
psychoaffectif
basketball
un compte-goutte
entretemps
six-cent-vingt-huit
un millefeuille
un portéclé

♦ Exercice récapitulatif 2 (p. 95)

Règles C
juger à priori
dérèglementation
faciès
crèmerie
cèleri
ambigüité
une voix aigüe
un yéti
indument
assèchement
un boitier
un client sélect
ils libèreraient

♦ Exercice récapitulatif 3 (p. 117)

Règles A à D
il parait
extrasensoriel
des lave-vaisselles
corolaire
une réponse ambigüe

interpeler
cent-cinquante
nivèlement
gastroentérite

évènement
cachotier
des habits chics
frisoter

♦ Exercice récapitulatif 4 (p. 137)

Règles A à F
relai
téléenseignement
règlementaire
antiinflammatoire
un millepatte
des vadémécums

hydroélectricité
en argüant
des égos
révolver
des terrepleins
une boite
combattive

♦ Exercice récapitulatif 5 (p. 159)

Règles G
yukonais
des appareils monoblocs
téléférique
granite
une réunion intergroupe
fiord

cuillère
nirvana
dribler
emmental
plateforme
canyon
tanin

♦ Exercice récapitulatif 6 (p. 162)

Règles A à G
altéa
bélouga
globetrotteur
chichekébab

guilde
hachich
à capella
etcétéra
goulache

Corrigé des jeux

♦ Je me cultive : culture générale I (p. 118)

Définitions : 1b, 2b, 3b, 4a, 5a, 6b, 7c, 8b, 9a, 10a, 11a, 12b, 13b, 14a, 15b, 16a, 17a, 18c.

Ne pas confondre les réponses ci-dessus avec des mots semblables : 1a→**foxterrier** (soudé A4), 4b→**typhon**, 6a→**wapitis**, 7b→**le** *Credo* (mot latin, inchangé C4), 9b→**un limès** (accent C4), 10b→**des bossanovas** (soudé A4, pluriel régulier B2), 11b→**exigüe** (tréma déplacé C3), 15a→**girole** (D3), 17b→**barquerole** (D3).

♦ Je me cultive : culture générale II (p. 160)

Définitions : 1a (ne pas confondre avec 1c→**tocarde**), 2a, 3c, 4b, 5a, 6b, 7b, 8a, 9c.

Associations de sens : 10b→**yak**, 10c→**yéti**, 11a→**goulache**, 11b→**paélia**, 12a→**calife**, 12c→**sanscrit**, 13b→**persiffler**, 13c→**parafer**, 14a→**rapsodie**, 14b→**vilénie**, 15a→**bernard-l'ermite**, 15d→**bélouga**, 16a→**téléférage**, 16b→**téléférique**, 17b→**réfréner**, 17c→**asséner**, 18a→**cleptomane**, 18c→**riquiqui**.

♦ Autres jeux et examen final

Les corrigés du **mot caché**, du **Dictomanie**, de la **dictée** et de l'**examen final « Je m'évalue »** sont en ligne au : www.nouvelleorthographe.info/corrige.html.

Pour recevoir gratuitement de l'information
sur l'orthographe par messagerie électronique
ou une **trousse d'autoformation gratuite
avec vidéos**, voyez les menus à ce sujet sur
www.nouvelleorthographe.info

Résumé des règles

Ce résumé ne retient que l'essentiel des règles. Pour les détails, voyez chacune des règles dans la section *Tests et exercices* de ce livre.

A   SOUDURE ET TRAIT D'UNION : SOUDURE...

A1 ...avec *contr(e)-* et *entr(e)-*

A2 ...avec *extra-, infra-, intra-, ultra-*

A3 ...dans les composés d'éléments savants

A4 ...dans les onomatopées et les emprunts

A5 ...dans plusieurs composés avec *-tout, bas(se)-, bien-, haut(e)-, mal-, mille-,* et dans quelques autres composés

A6   TRAIT D'UNION dans un numéral composé

B   SINGULIER et PLURIEL réguliers...

B1 ...dans les noms composés de type VERBE + NOM et aussi PRÉPOSITION + NOM

B2 ...dans les noms et adjectifs empruntés

C1   ACCENT GRAVE...

> é → è   avant une syllabe contenant « e muet »

...**dans des mots comme** *évènement, règlementaire, crèmerie, assèchement*

...**au futur et au conditionnel des verbes du type** *céder* (*cèdera, cèderait*)

...**dans les inversions avec** *-je* (*puissè-je*)

C2 ACCENT CIRCONFLEXE disparait sur *i* et *u*

| î → i | Exceptions : |

je crois, elle croit, nous partîmes/vous finîtes/qu'il fît...

| û → u | Exceptions : |

dû, mûr, sûr, jeûne(s), crûs/crût, eûmes/qu'il bût...

C3 TRÉMA déplacé

| -guë- → -güe- | (*ambigüe*)

| -guï- → -güi- | (*ambigüité*)

TRÉMA ajouté

| arguer → argüer | (*j'argüe*)

| -geure → -geüre | (*gageüre*)

C4 ACCENTS FRANÇAIS sur les emprunts

D CONSONNE SIMPLE

D1
| -elle → -èle (verbes en *-eler*) |

Exceptions : *appeler* et sa famille

| -ellement → -èlement (dérivés) |

| -ette → -ète (verbes en *-eter*) |

Exceptions : *jeter* et sa famille

| -ettement → -ètement (dérivés) |

D2 Consonne simple (et non double) après le son « e » (*interpeler, prunelier*)

| **D3** | **-olle → -ole** (et dérivés de ces mots) |

Exceptions : *colle, folle, molle*

| **-otter → -oter** (et dérivés de ces verbes) |

E Le participe passé *LAISSÉ* suivi d'un infinitif est invariable

F1 Quelques familles de mots sont harmonisées (*boursouffler, combattif*)

F2 Quelques anomalies sont supprimées (*exéma, levreau, ognon, nénufar, relai*)

| **F3** | **e → é** si l'accent aigu manquait (mot français) |

| **e → è** si l'accent grave manquait (mot français) |

| **F4** | **-illier → -iller** si le 2ᵉ **i** ne s'entend pas |

| **-illière → -illère** si le 2ᵉ **i** ne s'entend pas |

G Recommandations générales (si deux formes attestées coexistent en concurrence)

G1 à G20 → choisir la forme la plus

simple, française, non ambigüe
(*canyon, fiord, iglou, shampoing, granite*…)

G21 | **-er** (ou **-eur**) → **-eur** (francisation) |

G22 | → tenir compte d'innovations reconnues |

G23/G24 | 📖 **Néologismes** (pour les lexicographes) |

Pour les détails des règles G1 à G24, voir p. 140-141.

Bibliographie

Lectures recommandées

Connaitre et maitriser la nouvelle orthographe : guide pratique et exercices, de C. Contant et R. Muller, éd. De Champlain S. F., 2009 (*guide complet pour les professionnels, voir p. 193*).

Les rectifications de l'orthographe du français, de C. Contant et R. Muller, éd. ERPI et De Boeck, 2010 (*guide simplifié accessible, en couleurs, pour les non-spécialistes, voir p. 194-195*).

Grand vadémécum de l'orthographe moderne recommandée, de C. Contant, éd. De Champlain S. F., 2009 (*liste la plus complète, explications détaillées sur chaque mot, voir p. 200*).

Nouvelle orthographe : la liste simplifiée, de C. Contant, éd. De Champlain S. F., 2010 (*liste de 4000 mots, format de poche, voir p. 200*).

www.nouvelleorthographe.info : positions officielles, règles, liste de dictionnaires à jour, etc.

www.orthographe-recommandee.info : divers documents des ministères de l'Éducation, logos de conformité, correcteurs informatiques, etc.

Bibliographie pour ce livre

Académie française. *Dictionnaire de l'Académie française*, 9e édition, tome 1 (A-Enz) et tome 2 (Eoc-Map), éditions Fayard, Paris, 2000-2005.

Antidote RX (2009) et Antidote HD (2010), logiciel, Druide informatique, Montréal [www.druide.com].

CATACH, Nina, avec la coll. de J.-C. Rebejkow. *Varlex : variation lexicale et évolution graphique du français actuel*, CILF, Paris, 2001.

Conseil supérieur de la langue française (France). « Les rectifications de l'orthographe — Rapport », publié au *Journal officiel,* Paris, 6 décembre 1990.

CONTANT, Chantal. *Grand vadémécum de l'orthographe moderne recommandée*, éditions De Champlain S. F., Montréal, 2009.

Dictionnaire d'orthographe et de difficultés du français, éd. Dictionnaires Le Robert, Paris, 2010.

Dictionnaire Hachette et *Dictionnaire Hachette Junior*, éditions Hachette Éducation, Paris, 2010.

Larousse des noms communs, dictionnaire, éditions Larousse, Paris, 2008.

Nouveau Littré (2006) et *Nouveau Petit Littré* (2009, livre de poche), dictionnaires, éd. Garnier, Paris.

Petit Larousse illustré, dictionnaire, éditions Larousse, Paris, 1988 et 2010.

Petit Robert : dictionnaire alphabétique et analogique de la langue française, éd. Dictionnaires Le Robert, Paris, 1990 (*Petit Robert 1*) et 2010 (*Nouveau Petit Robert*).

RENOUVO (Réseau pour la nouvelle orthographe du français). Règles sur le site www.renouvo.org.

Word (2007 et 2010), logiciel d'Office de Microsoft.

Table des matières

Défiez l'orthographe ! — 5
- 70 tests, exercices, jeux et des mots courants — 5
- Les difficultés orthographiques — 6
- Une orthographe recommandée — 7
- À vos marques, partez ! — 7

Tests et exercices — 9

Le trait d'union et la soudure – règles A — 10
- Tests intuitifs et exercices — 11
- Vrai ou Faux — 51

Le singulier et le pluriel – règles B — 54
- Tests intuitifs et exercices — 55
- Vrai ou Faux — 65
- Exercice récapitulatif 1 — **67**

Les accents et le tréma – règles C — 68
- Tests intuitifs et exercices — 69
- Vrai ou Faux — 91
- Exercice récapitulatif 2 — **95**

Les consonnes doubles – règles D — 96
- Tests intuitifs et exercices — 97
- Vrai ou Faux — 115
- Exercice récapitulatif 3 — **117**
- ★ Jeu : culture générale I — **118**

Les anomalies rectifiées – règles E et F — 120
- Tests intuitifs et exercices — 121
- Vrai ou Faux — 134
- ★ Jeu : mot caché — **136**
- Exercice récapitulatif 4 — **137**

Les choix recommandés – règles G — 138
- Tests intuitifs et exercices — 139
- Vrai ou Faux — 151

✶ Jeu : Dictomanie	**154**
Exercice récapitulatif 5	**159**
✶ Jeu : culture générale II	**160**
Exercice récapitulatif 6	**162**
✶ Jeu : dictée trouée	**163**
✓ **Examen final**	**164**

500 mots courants — **167**
Liste de 500 mots courants — 168

Les dictionnaires se mettent à jour — **185**
15 exemples dans 10 dictionnaires — 186

Précisions linguistiques — **188**
demi-, **mi-**, **semi-**, **quasi(-)** — 188
vice-, **ex-**, **sous-**, **non(-)** — 189
vingt et **cent** — 189
Noms propres — 189

Démêlez le vrai du faux — **190**
Oui, la nouvelle orthographe… — 190
Non, la nouvelle orthographe… — 190
Oui, on peut mélanger les deux — 191
Non, n'hésitez plus — 191

Informations pratiques — **192**
Réglez votre correcteur — 192
Livres et sites — 192
Informations gratuites — 192

Ouvrages sur l'orthographe — **193**

Réponses — **201**
Corrigé des tests intuitifs — 201
Corrigé des exercices récapitulatifs — 206
Corrigé des jeux — 208

Résumé des règles — **209**

Bibliographie — **212**

Contes éducatifs

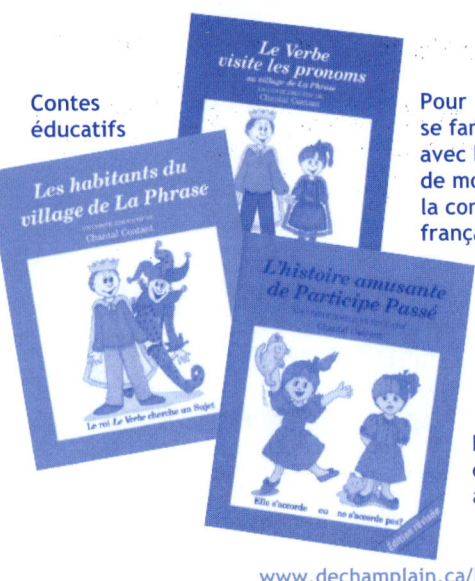

Pour se familiariser avec les classes de mots et la conjugaison française

En librairie en Europe et au Canada

www.dechamplain.ca/livres

Guide complet et exercices

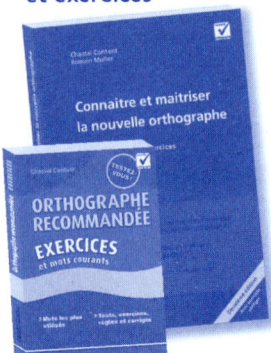

Listes de mots

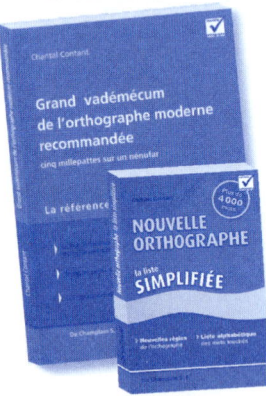